# BORG'S PERCEIVED EXERTION AND PAIN SCALES

## Gunnar Borg

Professor Emeritus of Perception and Psychophysics
Stockholm University

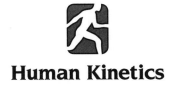

**Human Kinetics**

**Library of Congress Cataloging-in-Publication Data**

Borg, Gunnar.
   [Perceived exertion and pain scales]
   Borg's Perceived exertion and pain scales / Gunnar Borg.
      p.    cm.
   Includes bibliographical references and index.
   ISBN 0-88011-623-4
    1. Fatigue--Measurement.   2. Pain--Measurement.   3. Psychometrics.
  4. Medicine, Psychosomatic.  I. Title.
  QP321.B69   1998
  612'.044--dc21                           97-46439
                                          CIP

ISBN: 0-88011-623-4

**Acquisitions Editor:** Becky Lane; **Developmental Editor:** Julie Rhoda; **Assistant Editors:** Sandra Merz Bott and Cassandra Mitchell; **Editorial Assistant:** Laura T. Seversen; **Copyeditor:** Karen Bojda; **Proofreader:** Pam Johnson; **Indexer:** Craig Brown; **Graphic Designer:** Robert Reuther; **Cover Designer:** Jack Davis; **Illustrator:** Craig Ronto; **Printer:** United Graphics

Printed in the United States of America    10  9  8  7  6  5  4  3  2  1

**Human Kinetics**
Web site: http://www.humankinetics.com/

*United States:* Human Kinetics, P.O. Box 5076, Champaign, IL 61825-5076
1-800-747-4457
e-mail: humank@hkusa.com

*Canada:* Human Kinetics, Box 24040, Windsor, ON N8Y 4Y9
1-800-465-7301 (in Canada only)
e-mail: humank@hkcanada.com

*Europe:* Human Kinetics, P.O. Box IW14, Leeds LS16 6TR, United Kingdom
(44) 1132 781708
e-mail: humank@hkeurope.com

*Australia:* Human Kinetics, 57A Price Avenue, Lower Mitcham, South Australia 5062
(088) 277 1555
e-mail: humank@hkaustralia.com

*New Zealand:* Human Kinetics, P.O. Box 105-231, Auckland 1
(09) 523 3462
e-mail: humank@hknewz.com

# Contents

# *Preface*

This book contains information about methods for measuring subjective somatic symptoms. The main focus is on the presentation of two scaling methods: the Borg RPE scale and the Borg CR10 scale. The Borg RPE scale is a scale for ratings of perceived exertion (RPE). It is a tool for estimating effort and exertion, breathlessness, and fatigue during physical work. The Borg CR10 scale is a category-ratio (CR) scale anchored at the number 10, which represents extreme intensities. It is a general intensity scale for most subjective magnitudes that with special anchors can be used to measure exertion and pain.

A basic foundation for this book is the acceptance of a human as a psychosomatic whole. This means that psychological factors, such as personality, psychosocial factors, fear, and anxiety, affect somatic responses. It also means, however, that somatic functioning and signs of diseases can be studied psychologically, using human perception as a diagnostic instrument. This book deals primarily with the latter aspect.

Interest in perceived exertion, difficulty, health, and pain i.e., the subjective aspects of how we adapt to life, "how we are," has increased during the last decades. To feel well, be in good health, and feel alert and happy is a goal in itself. These feelings, and their unpleasant opposites (e.g., aches and pains, strain, and dissatisfaction), are important subjective cues that help us to react correctly and protect ourselves, as well as to act positively to improve our life situation. The sensory organs give important information of outer and inner conditions concerning both objects and events in the environment and reactions in the body.

Humans are built for physical work, but either too much or too little exercise can be detrimental. It is important to recognize an appropriate intensity level. In modern society, life's demands are more mental than physical. Our prehistoric, ancestral "fight and flight" response to stress is no longer a meaningful approach to problem solving. In the face of new situations and experiences, we must learn to act meaningfully and strongly enough in accordance with all relevant, integrated information. Thus, we also need a simple method to help us perceive and attend to important cues and their magnitudes in order to properly regulate our behavior.

The physical work we have to do or the exercise we should do to maintain good health always results in some degree of physical exertion. During hard physical work lasting several minutes, the demands on the heart, lungs, and working muscles are great. Because the heart has to work hard, heart rate (HR) is a common measure of degree of exertion. However, our own perceived exertion can also provide a good measure of physical exertion and intensity of exercise. When we exercise very hard, we feel it throughout our entire body. Breathlessness becomes annoying, and we feel the fatigue in our muscles. If these feelings become unpleasant, we may want to stop exercising. If, on the other hand, physical exertion is very light, we may feel no fatigue or discomfort, but rather a certain degree of well-being, such as that felt by many people during a nice walk. However, even an

> ## *Monitoring Effort in* Varpa
>
> A factor that was of special importance for my interest in the perceptions of effort and performance was my experience in childhood of *varpa* throwing (similar to throwing horse shoes). We often did that in our backyard using heavy, flat stones. It was astonishing to see how easily we could adjust our efforts so they were just right for the heaviness of the stone and the distance to the stick. Astonishingly, it was also possible to throw a different stone equally well; for example, if one stone cracked, you could throw another just as well. I made a small scientific study of this problem as an undergraduate in 1949 and confirmed the great discriminative ability of effort sensations and the possibility of transposition of psychomotor movement gestalt.

easy walk involves a certain degree of exertion, although very light.

Some physical activities may be so extreme, peculiar, or repetitive that they cause pain. This is not a major problem for healthy people but can be problematic in cases of pathology. In some situations pain is not caused by activities and distal stimulation but by an internal bodily disorder. The sensation of pain forces us to stop, listen, and try to understand the meaning of the messages and to cope with their implications immediately.

It may not be self-evident that a special method is needed for quantitative estimations and evaluations of subjective symptoms. In some situations qualitative judgments consisting of personal verbal expressions possibly may be useful and may fulfill the purpose at hand. Most often, however, it is necessary to have a defined method, a special scale constructed to facilitate comparisons of perceptual responses given by different people at different occasions and in different situations. This is the case when valid information is needed during an exercise test in a clinical setting or sports club. It is also of great value in training programs for the person on the street, athletes, or rehabilitation patients (e.g., people with cardiac diseases or musculoskeletal disorders). Finally, valid information is also needed for ergonomic and epidemiological evaluations of people at work or in the home.

Another reason for introducing a special methodology in this field is provided by the International Organization for Standardization (ISO). The ISO has stated that in efforts to improve work situations and tasks for men and women, both objective and subjective assessments must be taken into account. If subjective assessments are to play an important role, there must be a good

method that can be used in most situations and with most people.

The main purpose of the book is to introduce the field of perceived exertion and to present the commonly used Borg RPE scale and Borg CR10 scale with specific instructions, anchors, and explanations both for the test leader and for the person who is to respond using the scale; thus, the book can be used as a basic manual. At the moment no such manual is available since the only book about the Borg RPE scale was published more than 12 years ago (Borg 1985) and is now out of print. During the 12 years that have passed, the need for a good, basic manual that also gives examples of the many different situations in which scaling can or should be used has become evident.

The literature on pain is much more comprehensive than that on perceived exertion. The field of pain is also very old and has attracted the attention of many researchers and clinicians. Its importance in clinical diagnostics and therapy as well as in daily life and human communication is great. In spite of this, methods to evaluate pain intensity were rather poor until a few decades ago. As a matter of fact, the major progress was made after the introduction of the new psychophysics (S.S. Stevens 1957, 1975). Since one of the new methods for examining perceived exertion (and several other sensory modalities) is also well suited to assessment of pain intensity, I devote a great deal of space to problems of pain and show how the Borg CR10 scale is applicable to studies of both perceived exertion and pain.

The book gives information about the background of perceptual scaling (discussing its advantages and pitfalls), the construction and use of scaling methods, different situations in which scaling is important, and some physiological correlates to perception. The basic problems concern general psychological functioning—that is, common intraindividual reactions typical of all human beings—showing how the perceptual response varies with stimulation, particularly exercise intensity in well-controlled laboratory experiments. General studies of perceptual growth functions with a high degree of intersubjectivity (interindividual agreement) are then extended to psychophysiological comparisons in order to explain the appearance of the functions (using the physiological correlates as possible causes).

Problems of differences in general functions that vary with duration, frequency, and mode of exercise—for example, bicycling, running, or walking at different paces or variations of work tasks in manual materials handling—lead to other important areas of investigation. Added to this are the effects of environment, nutrition, drugs, and psychological factors such as attention and emotions.

All these basic, general problems also have their differential (interindividual) counterparts. Even if people react similarly in many fundamental ways, differences among individuals also exist, depending on age, sex, fitness, emotion, personality, and social context. Of special interest are the differential problems that can be attributed to rating behavior, emotion, and motivation. In addition are the individual differences resulting from specific diseases or more or less well-defined pathological factors.

This book is written for a wide audience including people interested in medicine, psychology, sports, ergonomics, and epidemiology. Because the book is intended for such a wide audience, it focuses on methodology. As for other basic methods in physiology—for example, measuring oxygen consumption ($\dot{V}O_2$), heart rate (HR), or lactate concentration—the Borg RPE scale and the Borg CR10 scale may be used in many diagnostic situations to help as-

sess symptoms of clinical relevance, estimate working capacity, help people monitor exercise intensities, select or adapt work tasks in manual materials handling, evaluate effects of therapy and rehabilitation, and evaluate intensities of daily life activities in epidemiological health investigations.

Most people interested in the field of perceived exertion are also interested in the field of pain. This is not only natural, but also necessary, since perceived exertion and pain—the most important subjective somatic symptoms that are provoked by heavy physical work—may overlap a great deal. However, perceived exertion is caused mainly by exercise (except for some minor sensory "noise" at rest, e.g., slight feelings of fatigue or breathlessness), while pain at rest commonly results from disease or injuries.

The broad scope of this book and the general usefulness of the methods should make it interesting for many kinds of doctors, nurses, physiotherapists, and exercise supervisors, both researchers and those who are clinically oriented and working in the fields of exercise physiology, the psychophysiology of stress and health, cardiology, pulmonary diseases, musculoskeletal disorders, dietetics, pain, ergonomics, biotechnology, and epidemiology. Coaches, professional or amateur athletes, or anyone with a profound interest in sports and exercise should also find the book useful.

This is not an exhaustive textbook. Not all of the many different situations or examples in which scaling is or can be used are included here. The purpose is to present the theoretical background, the methods, their applications, and some representative empirical examples. I have devoted much space to scale construction as well as to the reliability and validity of the Borg RPE scale and the Borg CR10 scale. I have also included a section on administering the scales and invite you to use this book as a manual for proper testing.

# Acknowledgments

I was glad when I had decided to start writing this book. At that time I had not realized that it could be such hard work. I am therefore very happy now that it is finished, and I want to thank my wife, Yvonne, for her wonderful understanding and support, and my daughter Elisabet for her great help, both in important research (including many creative ideas) and in all stages of the publication process. Thanks also to my son for taking part in some experiments and good discussions, to Ms. Karen A. Williams for helping me correct some of the English, and to the editors at Human Kinetics for all their help.

# PART I

# *Overview and History*

# Chapter 1

## Perceived Exertion

The psychophysiology of perceived exertion is a field partly within psycho physics, the scientific field that deals with measuring sensory perception. The main subfields in psychophysics are detection, identification, discrimination, and scaling, and of these, scaling is most important for the field of perceived exertion. When I started to study psychology in the mid-1940s, scaling was not a large field. At that time there were no good methods for scaling, and theories and applications were lacking. The idea of using the human sensory system as an instrument for measuring somatic symptoms hardly existed.

## Developing the Concept

The concept of perceived exertion was introduced at the end of the 1950s, together with methods for measuring overall perceived exertion, local fatigue, and breathlessness, and it was soon followed by several scientific studies and clinical, sports-related, and ergonomic applications. The field is now rather large; each year more than 200 scientific articles in this area are published, and in America alone about one million people are exposed to the methods of rating perceived exertion each year.

The concept of perceived exertion emanated from the first problem formulations and pilot studies by Borg and Dahlström in the 1950s. The content and meaning of perceived exertion are primarily given by common sense, personal experiences, and empirical studies. Experiences such as effort, breathlessness, fatigue, aches in the working muscles, feelings of warmness, and so on help to capture the concept. Other related concepts are subjective weight and heaviness, subjective force, arousal, and exercise intensity.

What we commonly feel and describe as fatigue has much in common with perceived exertion. During, or just after, heavy physical exercise, the meanings of fatigue and perceived exertion are very similar. There are, however, some important differences between the two concepts. *Fatigue* refers to a state that might be called "drowsiness," or a high level of tiredness or exhaustion. In this state, an individual's performance capacity has diminished. As a matter of fact, the term *fatigue* is often used in situations "where a transient decrease of working capacity results from previous physical activity" (Asmussen 1979). Fatigue is, thus, often defined physiologically or in relation to decrements in performance rather than in perceptual terms.

The perception of *exertion* (and effort), on the other hand, at very high intensities is also connected with diminishing working capacity, but at low or moderate intensities may be related to a state of activation, an "arousal" that has a positive effect on performance. Studying fatigue and exertion only from a physiological perspective is as impossible as dealing with color, emotion, or motivation in primarily physical or only physiological terms. That is, exertion and fatigue are states with both physiological and psychological aspects.

A concept related to fatigue and exertion is *exercise intensity*. Exercise intensity is interpreted several different ways. It may be given a physical, stimulus-based meaning, defined by physical measurements such as power, work and energy, torque, velocity, and so on. It may also be interpreted physiologically, in absolute terms such as $\dot{V}O_2$ or by relative values such as heart rate (HR). A third possibility is to evaluate exercise intensity in terms of ratings of subjective intensity as perceived by the subject. The latter method gives an individualized measure of exercise intensity directly.

The perception of exertion may be looked upon as a kind of *gestalt*, or configuration of sensations: strain, aches, and fatigue from the peripheral muscles and the pulmonary system, and some other sensory cues (Borg 1962a). When performing a heavy muscular task, we receive sensations from the muscles and joints, from somatosensory receptors, from the cardiovascular and respiratory systems, and from other bodily organs. Thus, many physiological cues are involved, as well as memories of work situations and actual performances and the emotions associated with them. The special situation in which work is performed may emphasize certain aspects of it, suppressing some sensations and making the subject attend to and concentrate on other sensations. Motivation and emotions during the exercise may also influence perception and performance.

Another concept related to perceived exertion, fatigue, and exercise intensity is *dangerous strain*. Some subjective somatic symptoms, especially during heavy exercise, may be signs of disease (e.g., angina pain, difficulty in breathing [dyspnea]) rather than of exertion, fatigue, or strong local pain in the musculoskeletal system. It is important for an exercising individual to pay attention to such symptoms and to be able to distinguish them from normal perceived exertion. This is not always easy, particularly because some symptoms or signs may be silent and impossible to perceive. A physical examination by a clinical specialist is therefore always recommended at regular intervals.

It is of great theoretical as well as practical interest to identify the different physiological components involved in physical exertion and to find out how they vary in relation to perceived exertion. To explain the variance across subjects and workloads, we must measure many different physiological variables, decide how to weigh them, study their interactions, and try to develop a statistical model for predictions. However, when this is done, the difficulty is just beginning. We must also collect data about each individual's mental reactions: cognitive, motivational, and emotional functioning; personality traits and states; and his or her "rating behavior." We must, of course, have very reliable and valid methods

in order to measure all these variables. To further complicate the task, we must also understand the given work situation and environment in which the subject is exercising. Thus, we must ultimately understand the person-by-situation interaction! So, it would seem that the task of statistically explaining and understanding the perceived exertion process through research is very difficult and cannot be dealt with by the present state of the art. It is, however, a great challenge for further research!

Ten years ago at a meeting about exercise intensity that I attended, a physiologist was asked if he had recorded any perceptual responses. The physiologist answered that he had not been interested in psychic problems or mental stress but in physical exertion. His answer is of great interest, since it reveals a misunderstanding that is still rather common: that physical load has to be studied using only physiological measurements. In psychology it is common to study mental load by using both physiological stress responses (such as catecholamine excretion) and mental responses (such as perceived exertion or difficulty). Figure 1.1 elucidates this problem.

The degree of effective physical strain (exertion) behind a performance is sometimes difficult to measure, especially in cases where a pathology is present. Dangerous strain may therefore be looked upon as a hypothetical construct, an inner state or event that may be difficult to identify, like a submarine. It is there, of course, and good evidence of its existence may be obtained from both subjective and objective indicators, either of which may be incomplete or misleading when taken by itself. It is therefore important to try to integrate as many different kinds of symptoms and signs as possible.

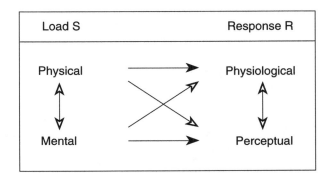

**Figure 1.1** Both physiological and perceptual responses should be used as indicators of physical and mental workload.

# Early Perceived Exertion Studies

Within academic psychology in the 1940s many discussions took place about different schools, such as psychoanalysis, gestalt psychology, behaviorism, and learning theory. General and experimental psychology were rather popular, and laboratories often smelled of rats. Differential psychology was growing fast, and psychometric methods were being refined. There had been many applications of psychometric methods for selection of personnel during World War II and later for vocational guidance; human factors and ergonomics helped to improve instruments and work tasks. Clinical psychology focused on diagnostic tools for personality disorders, and very few researchers were engaged in preventive medicine and health care. There was only weak contact between academic psychology and applied psychology. In spite of the old academic tradition in experimental psychology and psychophysics, there was little interest among clinical psychologists in using the theories and tools from sensory perception and psychophysics to study complaints and subjective somatic symptoms.

Psychophysical studies by S.S. Stevens and collaborators at Harvard (Stevens 1957, 1971; Stevens and Galanter 1957) showed that sensory perception often does not grow linearly with physical stimulation but according to positively or negatively accelerating power functions (see S.S. Stevens 1975). Thus the perception of loudness follows a negatively accelerating function with an exponent of about 0.6 and the sensation of an electric shock follows a positively accelerating one with an exponent of about 3.0. Therefore, depending on the kind of stimulation and the sensory modality involved, a given increase in physical stimulation may cause an increase in sensory perception that deviates a great deal from the physical one. If the physical increase is 100%, the perceptual one may be 200% or only 50%.

At the end of the 1950s I had started a psychophysical study on the perception of speed while driving a car (Borg 1961c; see also Borg 1962a). The study had shown that perception of speed grows with the square of the physical speed. The idea was then put forth that the perception of exertion during physical exercise might follow a similar "distorted" growth function. This would then mean that a lumber worker's experience of a decline in working capacity of 50% could possibly correspond to a physical decrease of only 30%. The argument behind this idea was the following: People do not directly perceive a decline in working capacity, but rather an increase in exertion. If it used to feel easy to work in the garden or walk up four flights of stairs in an apartment building but it now feels twice as hard, it may be reasonable to estimate that the working

---

## Perceived Exertion: How It All Started

The first studies of perceived exertion were inspired by a discussion about the possible relationships between an individual's subjective judgment of his or her working capacity and objective measurements of the capacity. During the spring semester of 1958, at the medical school in Umeå, Sweden, I was teaching psychology and Hans Dahlström, head of the laboratory for clinical physiology, was teaching physiology. During a coffee break, Hans and I started to discuss problems related to fatigue and working capacity. Hans told me about his patients and their experiences of working capacity and fatigue and how they were related to results from tests on the bicycle ergometer. Sometimes the individual's own evaluation of his or her working capacity did not agree well with the test value as shown by the ergometer. A middle-aged lumberjack, for example, could complain that his working capacity had gone down by 50%, while a clinical examination might reveal a decrease of only half as much. This lack of correspondence undermined communication between the doctor and the patient. Sometimes the patient was suspected of fabricating a decreased working capacity in order to gain insurance or retirement benefits; however, investigation in greater detail rarely unveiled any such deceptions. The decrease in working capacity is not perceived directly but estimated indirectly from the increase in perceived exertion. A preliminary hypothesis was then put forth that the subject's judgment might be "distorted" due to a general "error" in the perceptual process.

capacity has gone down to half of what it was before. However, that presupposes a linear relationship between changes in perceived exertion for physical exercise and changes in working capacity. But if a linear relationship is not the case—if perceived exertion follows a function similar to that for perception of speed while driving a car—then misjudgments of decrements in working capacity can be understood and predicted.

Studies by Borg and Dahlström were thus started in Sweden in 1958. These studies did not concern experiences of or changes in working capacity per se, but rather addressed the issue of perceived exertion and its variation as a function of changes in physical workload. The first studies dealt with perceptual judgments of effort and pedal resistance during short-duration (seconds or a few minutes) exercise on a bicycle ergometer (Borg and Dahlström 1959, 1960) and then during work of longer duration (several or many minutes) and work of differential and clinical interest (Borg 1962a; Borg and Linderholm 1967).

Prior to these studies, there had been some experiments on perceptual aspects of fatigue in relation to physiological variables, but no real psychophysical scaling methods were used. Fatigue, in a broad sense, is an old field in terms of both research and application. Early studies of effort and fatigue had been done in industrial settings; many of these were work studies or time studies. One of the first fatigue scales was Poffenberger's 7-point rating scale from 1928, which was designed to obtain ratings of workers' feelings of fatigue (Poffenberger 1928). Other studies on the perception of fatigue did not measure the variations in intensity as scaling experiments do, but only tried to classify some intensity levels or to describe them semantically (see Bartley and Chute 1945).

Studies on the perception of heaviness when lifting weights have been part of laboratory studies since Weber and Fechner did their fundamental experiments in the 19th century (Fechner 1860). Most studies of subjective weight, however, have not dealt with scaling of perceived exertion in hard work, but with establishing thresholds when lifting rather light cans.

No psychophysical studies were carried out earlier because methods for such scaling were not developed until the 1950s by S.S. Stevens (1957). These psychophysical ratio scaling methods started a new area of research in psychology and psychophysiology. Most attributes of sensory perceptions and experiences were studied using these scaling methods (see S.S. Stevens 1975). Fatigue in the sense of perceived exertion, however, was not studied until we started the new research projects in Sweden at the end of the 1950s.

Other factors also allowed the field of perceived exertion to be opened up. In the 1950s, the development of reliable ergometers in exercise laboratories and hospitals and in clinical testing was an important advancement. The need to understand people's perceptions better and to integrate information from subjective symptoms

## Why on Earth Should This Be of Interest?

A question that I sometimes am asked is how the first studies were received, how the interest started to grow, and how strong it is now. The answer is that the first studies were rather well received among both scientists and clinicians. In Sweden psychologists were interested in psychophysical scaling, and medical doctors and physiologists were interested in clinical and ergonomic applications. In most other countries, including the United States, interest in scaling was not as great, however, except for a few scientists at Harvard working with S.S. Stevens and his colleagues. After my dissertation was published in 1962 (Borg 1962a), I was very glad to receive a letter from Stevens in which he congratulated me for having opened up a new field for psychophysical research. However, there were quite a few who didn't like Stevens's ratio scaling methods. I remember that when I was in Philadelphia and gave a talk at the Department of Psychology during the spring of 1968, an elderly professor asked me: "Why on earth do you think this should be of interest?" I was very puzzled and not prepared to give a good answer. I said something about there being many interesting theoretical and methodological problems and applications, but I don't think I convinced him that my research was either interesting or important. In 1980, 12 years later, however, perceived exertion had obviously become one of the biggest fields within applied psychophysics.

with physiological signs also became more and more apparent and forced a development in this direction.

An important factor that contributed to the development of studies in perceived exertion in the United States was the invitation I received in 1967 to visit B. Noble in Pittsburgh and E. Buskirk, J. Skinner, and O. Bar-Or at State College, Pennsylvania (see Borg and Noble 1974). Several laboratory experiments were performed in the 1960s and 1970s by Noble and several of his students (among others, Cafarelli, Metz, Pandolf, Robertson, and Stamford; see Noble and Borg 1972), then by several others in the United States, and by Onodera and Miyashita in Japan in 1976. In Holland, Hueting (1965) performed experiments on sensations of general physical fatigue, which were independent of our work. Clinical studies of perceived exertion in the United States became more common in the 1970s, owing much to Pollock and his collaborators (see Gutman et al. 1981), and perceived exertion in connection with personality studies became another field of interest thanks to Morgan (1973).

Subjective force of hand grip is another related field; the first studies of this topic were performed by J.C. Stevens and Mach (1959) at the same time as we (Borg and Dahlström [1959]) independently started experiments in perceived exertion. They used direct ratio scaling methods and obtained positively accelerating stimulus-response (S-R) functions that were similar to ours, that is, with exponents around 1.7. A critical difference between our studies on perceived exertion and the subjective force of hand grip studies, however, was that the latter studies did not involve heavy exercise with big muscles, exercise that stresses the cardiovascular and respiratory systems. A special development of the studies of subjective force was in cross-modal matching (the CMM method), whereby perceptual intensities in one modality (e.g., loudness) can be measured by "matches" (e.g., equal settings or ratio settings) in another modality (e.g., subjective force of hand grip; see S.S. Stevens 1975).

Our first studies, on the other hand, focused mainly on overall perceived exertion and the two major components involved:

1. The sensations of pressure, subjective force, strain, and fatigue originating from the somatosensory system and the muscles engaged in executing the performance (perceived pedal resistance and aches in the legs)

2. The exertion from the chest originating from the cardiopulmonary system (panting or breathlessness; Borg 1961b, 1962a)

The importance of these two components was then stressed by Ekblom and Goldberg (1971) who coined the terms *local* and *central* perceived exertion. Noble and his co-workers in Pittsburgh then did several significant studies of these factors and their relative contribution to overall perceived exertion; especially notable are the studies by Pandolf, Burse, and Goldman (1975), and Robertson et al. (1979). Weiser and Stamper (1977) identified the dimensions *general fatigue* and *leg fatigue,* and then an emotional component, which they labeled *task aversion.*

# The Three Effort Continua

In physical and mental work it is often important to try to integrate results from the three main *effort continua:* the perceptual, the performance, and the physiological (Borg 1977). Figure 1.2 illustrates these three effort continua. In this figure, O denotes the subject or "observer" who is performing a certain physical task, S. The goal is to try to identify different levels or zones of subjective intensities, for example, adaptation or preference levels, training zones, and stress levels. In psychophysical studies the interest has focused on relative growth functions but not on important levels of intensity that can be applied to real-life situations. This has been a great drawback and delayed the answers to fundamental questions such as the following:

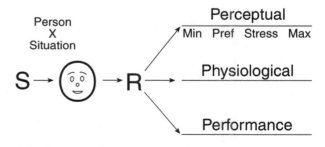

**Figure 1.2**   The three effort continua: perceptual, performance, and physiological. S is the stimulus that interacts with the situation and the person (the observer, O). R is the response in each of these continua. The intensity varies in all continua from minimum (Min) over other levels (such as a preferred or adaptation level [Pref] and a stress level [Stress]) to maximal (Max) intensity.

- What is the intensity level at which a subject prefers to work?
- What is the perceived exertion for most people when training at an appropriate intensity for cardiac rehabilitation?
- To what level may a person have to adapt in doing daily work? (If the daily adaptation level is too close to a maximal intensity, the person will be stressed and the cost of the work will be too great.)

## Perceptual Continuum

It is natural for a psychologist to start the inquiry and the investigations from the perceptual continuum since perception plays a fundamental role in our behavior and in how we adapt to a situation. From a theoretical point of view the perceptual continuum is also fundamental since the meaning of a concept often has to start from a person's subjective experience. To study stress and strain we must start to identify the problem by asking people about their experiences of stressful situations and responses. These subjective aspects must have an epistemic priority to be meaningful. By this I mean that in this context the subjective aspect is a fundamental basis in the theory of knowledge and should be given priority in this scientific inquiry.

There is a corresponding performance continuum and a corresponding physiological continuum. For each continuum there are different levels or zones in the other continua. Since these three continua are not interrelated in a simple and linear way, however, we cannot just translate values from one to the other, but must study each specifically and try to integrate the data.

## Performance Continuum

Performances that are easiest to define, and sometimes also to measure (though not in pathological cases), are maximal performances, such as the highest workload ($W_{max}$) a subject can manage for a certain amount of time, using workload as the dependent variable and keeping time constant, such as 30 s for Borg's Cycling Strength Test (CST; Borg 1982b). Other performance measures are the shortest time in which a subject can run a mile or the longest distance a subject can run for 12 min (the Cooper Test; Cooper 1968). Submaximal performances, such as preferred intensity levels, are also possible to determine.

Specific psychomotor performances such as reaction time and hand-arm trembling belong to another class of performances. These kinds of performances are quite different from the simpler muscular performances, and they vary with intensity in a different way than do muscular performances and physiological variables. They are, however, also sensitive to physical exertion and do thus indicate the degree of exertion, especially trembling.

## Physiological Continuum

The physiological continuum includes many variables such as HR, $\dot{V}O_2$, blood and muscle lactate, ventilation and respiration rates, and catecholamine excretion, to name just a few. In contrast to the variables belonging to the perceptual continuum, physiological functions are rather easy to measure using physical methods. The growth functions of the operationally defined physiological variables have different appearances; some (e.g., $\dot{V}O_2$ and HR) are linearly related to the stimulus intensity measured, for example, in watts, while others (e.g., positively accelerating functions such as lactate concentration) show nonlinear increases. Even if the physiological responses are rather easy to measure, it is not so easy to know how to integrate and give weight to the variables in order to best predict performance. The perception of exertion may facilitate a solution to this problem in some situations, since overall perception integrates many cues from all over the body and automatically (and intuitively) gives special weight to the most important ones.

The three effort continua—the perceptual, the performance, and the physiological—complement each other. They give partly different information, and the variables belonging to them are not all linearly related to each other. An exercise intensity of 50% of maximal working capacity may thus correspond to a 45% increase in one variable but only 30% in another. To obtain a valid and complete picture of an individual's exertion, it is important to collect and integrate all available information from all three effort continua.

Figure 1.3 shows six hypothetical frequency distributions of exercise intensities on these effort continua. Most exercise intensities are weak, and the extremely hard intensities are rare and mainly found in athletic competitions and special maximal and lactate training programs. The minimal (Min) and maximal (Max) intensities are

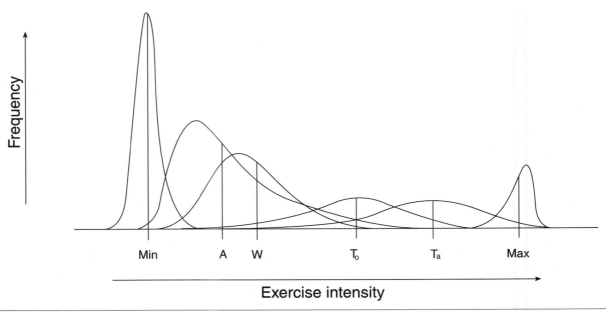

**Figure 1.3** Hypothetical examples of frequency distributions for some common levels of exercise intensity from minimum to maximum. A stands for activities of daily life (ADL), W for manual work, T for training intensity for ordinary people ($T_o$) and for athletes ($T_a$). The positions and sizes of the distributions will vary with mode and duration of exercise.

not absolute, exact levels but vary to some degree. In figure 1.3 the distribution around A refers to activities of daily life (ADL) during ordinary leisure-time activities (with no special physical training involved), W to heavy physical work (e.g., in physically demanding occupational work), and T to special exercise and training (with aerobic training at about 40% to 80% of maximum). Measurements of these intensities may be obtained from performances, from physiological responses, and from ratings of perceptual intensities.

# Defining Perceived Exertion

All the related and subordinate concepts described in the preceding sections help us specify a constitutional definition of the concept of perceived exertion. The concept mainly refers to heavy muscular work involving a relatively great strain on the musculoskeletal, cardiovascular, and pulmonary systems. Perceived exertion is thus closely related to the concept of exercise intensity. At the same time, special motivational, emotional, and pathological conditions may be involved in such a way that the concept broadens to include additional, if less dominant, factors.

This means that somewhat different content may be given to the concept of perceived exertion depending on the situation and context, the operational definition, and the method of exercise used.

This is a prominent constitutional definition: Perceived exertion is the feeling of how heavy and strenuous a physical task is. This definition emphasizes the physical strain experienced in muscular work. In most healthy subjects the focus is mainly on subjective aspects of stimulus intensity and the sensory experience of exercise. However, the strain experienced may also involve pain and affective components, reflecting special individual states and traits.

The constitutional definition is fundamental but does not give any direct measure of the degree of perceived exertion. For this, an operational definition is needed that anchors the concept to a measurable variable (or construct) based on a specific methodology. This means that a measure of perceived exertion is defined by the constitutional definition together with a scaling method and instruction for its use.

An interesting article on perceived exertion was published by P. Hage (1981). The article covered many important points but had a somewhat misleading title: "Perceived Exertion: One Measure of Exercise Intensity." To be correct it should have read "Ratings of Perceived Exertion"; perceived exertion itself is not a measure. Furthermore, for the rating to be a measure it must be operationally defined.

Ratings of perceived exertion (RPE) can be obtained in several ways, such as with the Borg RPE scale and the Borg CR10 scale. A measure of perceived exertion is the *degree of heaviness and strain experienced in physical work as estimated according to a specific rating method* (such as the Borg RPE scale).

The given definition of RPE refers to overall perceived exertion, which depends on many factors—sensory cues and somatic symptoms, emotional factors, rating behavior, and so on—integrated into a kind of gestalt or configuration. The different factors interact, and depending on the person and performance in question, some factors may intuitively be given special weight for the overall RPE value.

If some factors, such as local sensations of strain in the working muscles, dominate over others, the term *local RPE* (or leg RPE, arm RPE, etc.) is used. The term *chest RPE* is used if breath-lessness is the dominant sensation. I first proposed this division of perceived exertion (Borg 1961b, 1962a).

In exercise with small muscle groups or exercise of short duration (seconds), the local sensations dominate, while for heavy exercise during several minutes, chest exertion may dominate because of the strain on the cardiopulmonary system. Ekblom and Goldberg (1971) use the terms *local* and *central* perceived exertion to differentiate the two divisions; however, this terminology can be misleading because "central" in physiology refers mainly to reactions in the central nervous system.

Perceived exertion and pain are two concepts that partly overlap. During very heavy work some people, especially those with disease or illness, may get pain in the legs or chest. The psychophysical methods used when studying pain are the same as or similar to those used when studying perceived exertion. The next chapter, therefore, discusses pain.

# Chapter 2

## Pain

**P**ain is an old concept, and its general meaning is well understood by most people all over the world. There are, however, many different kinds of pain from different parts of the body, which result from different types of tissue damage or disease. The affective components may also differ quite a bit from situation to situation. Furthermore, a given expression of pain may depend more or less on cultural differences.

The meaning of pain is given primarily by each individual's subjective reactions, sensory perceptions, experiences, emotions, memories, and ideas. There are currently many good, objective physiological correlates to pain, but an individual's perception must have an epistemic priority; that is, individual, subjective perception must be the starting point for studies and interpretations of pain.

Throughout human history, pain has certainly been one of the most fundamental concepts and a matter of great interest in a countless number of daily situations. However, methods for obtaining reliable estimates of pain perception were principally lacking until the 1960s. Before that, rather simple rating scales were used—and in some cases are still used, especially in clinical settings. These rank-order scales did not permit any real quantitative evaluations of changes in pain (Price 1988).

The ratio scaling methods introduced by S.S. Stevens (1957) gave researchers tools to measure perceptual intensities in most modalities, including pain. However, problems in providing, varying, and controlling distal or proximal stimulus intensities, including good techniques for anchoring standard intensities, delayed methodological development. An additional problem confronting researchers concerned interpreting a response and separating the sensory from the affective or cognitive part of the response.

My own interest in pain assessment followed the studies of perceived exertion. In laboratory experiments most healthy subjects could work very hard (on a bicycle ergometer) without symptoms of pain. When the subjects interrupted a test at voluntary maximum, they did not do this because of great pain but because of perceived exertion, breathlessness, or fatigue in the legs. The latter symptom was sometimes described as "aches" in the legs, but this ache was not pain of the kind caused by noxious stimulation. It is otherwise common in psychophysical experiments that an increase of the stimulus has to be interrupted at very high intensities because the sensation changes its quality, turning into pain. This is evident in one's perception of loudness, heat, cold, touch, and taste, for example.

At the same time that we performed the first laboratory studies on perceived exertion in healthy subjects, we also studied hospital patients' perception of exertion. Scaling perceived exertion soon became routine during clinical stress tests. In many pathological cases, such as in patients with coronary insufficiencies and angina pain or with musculoskeletal disorders, the quality of perceived exertion changed during the test because of pain, and the test had to be interrupted (see Borg 1962a; Borg and Linderholm 1970; Borg, Holmgren, and Lindblad 1981). The need for a special scale that could be used for perceived exertion but also for other sensory perceptions, including pain, became more and more evident and several methodological studies were initiated that finally led to the Borg CR10 scale (Borg 1982b; Borg, Holmgren, and Lindblad 1981).

# Defining Pain

Since pain is such an old and well-established concept (Merskey [1991] gives a basic definition), the dictionaries give constitutional definitions of primarily the same kind or content in most languages. *The Shorter Oxford Universal Dictionary* (Onions 1968) gives the definition: "The opposite of pleasure; the sensation which one feels when hurt (in body or mind); suffering, distress. . . . Bodily suffering; a distressing sensation as of soreness (usually in a particular part of the body). . . . Mental suffering; trouble, grief, sorrow." *The American Heritage Dictionary of the English Language* (Morris 1969) defines pain as "an unpleasant sensation, occurring in varying degrees of severity as a consequence of injury, disease, or emotional disorder. . . . Suffering or distress."

The International Association for the Study of Pain (IASP) defines pain as "an unpleasant sensory and emotional experience associated with actual or potential tissue damage, or described in terms of such damage" (Merskey and Bogduk 1994). This definition implicates both sensory (i.e., nociception) and emotional (i.e., suffering) factors. It also draws on both "actual" and "potential" events. This definition is now questioned; there is a proposal that it should be broadened to include other aspects of pain communication (Anand and Craig 1996).

The general usage and the high degree of intersubjectivity make the concept of pain very useful to most people. However, even if most people use the word *pain* in about the same way, there are still some differences due to personal experience and culture. This is especially true of the meaning of degrees of pain when making interindividual comparisons. Also, when it comes to qualities of pain, there are differences depending on the extent to which special cognitive and emotional factors are involved. For example, your perception of chest pain may be different depending on whether you are very certain that the pain was caused by falling and hurting yourself or whether you think it is a symptom of heart failure.

Therefore, it is necessary in research and in many clinical situations to better define the kind of pain studied and what method is or should be used to measure the specific aspect of interest for a given person in a given situation. One way to do this is to define specific constructs of pain that are firmly dependent on the method and instruction used. For instance, a patient with cardiovascular disorders and local pain in the legs resulting from *claudicatio intermittence* (a circulatory disorder) should give an estimate of the degree of aches and pain after a brisk walk of a certain distance (preferably also with controlled conditions, speed, and duration) using, for example, the Borg CR10 scale with specific instructions.

# Special Aspects of Pain

There are many classifications and many components of pain. Often acute damage of somatic or visceral tissue causes stimulation of nociceptors (pain receptors). This pain is often of an acute character and steady or recurrent depending on special activities and proximal stimulation. It may also be chronic if the damage is not healed or if there are other reasons for ongoing stimulation of the nociceptors. Even without an appreciable somatic reason for the pain, such as direct nociceptive stimulation, the pain may still be there, interacting with psychological factors, and may be idiopathic. Neurogenic pain is caused by damage to the peripheral or central nervous systems. If there is no clear somatic cause at all, the pain is often called psychogenic.

The expressions of different kinds of pain may overlap a great deal, because pain is not just a specific somatic symptom, such as a nociceptive

---

## *The Borg RPE Scale Is Alive and So Is Borg*

The Borg RPE scale has become a standard method in exercise testing, training, and rehabilitation. In some hospitals in Sweden it has been used for so many years that the nurses administering the test think that the scale dates back a generation. When my older brother was tested because of heart problems, the nurse instructed him about the use of the RPE scale. He remarked, "My younger brother constructed this scale." The nurse looked astonished and said, "Oh, is he still alive?"

pain related to a certain organ of the body, but a psychosomatic symptom, with physiological reactions that interact with an individual's mental functioning, personality, motivation, emotion, and cognitive factors. The meaning of the pain in a certain situation has to be interpreted specifically for each person in terms of the suffering it causes.

In determining the character of pain it is important to localize the pain's focus, extent, radiation, and time pattern. The pain may be sharp but last for only a few seconds or fractions of a second, or it may last for hours or months. Several kinds of pain may also happen at the same time: one a rather steady but weak background feeling and another a sharp sensation coming suddenly or intermittently. From patients' personal experiences it is sometimes possible to identify different kinds of pain as dull, twinging, cutting, pricking, tingling, shooting, numbing, cramping, and so on.

There are different physiological mechanisms related to the different kinds or time courses of pain, for example, cutaneous A-beta, A-delta, and C primary afferent fibers. Several biochemical substances are involved, such as neuropeptides, autocoids, histamine, hydrogen ions, and so on (Dray, Urban, and Dickenson 1994). A substance that we have studied in Stockholm is the adenosine that may provoke angina pectoris–like pain. A power function with a very high goodness of fit showing how pain increases with adenosine was obtained using the Borg CR10 scale (Sylvén et al. 1988).

The intensity of pain is most easily determined if the primary goal is to compare changes within a person, or responses of the same person before and after therapy. When there is a need to make "absolute" determinations of intensity levels and interindividual comparisons, the difficulties are much greater. This is also the case if pain is studied over a long period of time when cues for pain memories may fluctuate quite a bit.

While this book cannot detail and discuss every different kind of pain and its source, with the proper instructions, scaling pain and most perceptions using an intensity scale such as the CR10 scale is possible. The next chapter will help you learn how to measure perceived exertion and pain using my RPE and CR10 scales.

# Chapter 3

## Measuring Perceived Exertion and Pain

The general term for the scientific field that deals with theories and methods for measuring psychological processes is *psychometrics*. If we restrict the field to measurements of perceived intensities we talk of *psychophysics*, an old term that may be confusing for the layperson. The term *psychophysics* may be mistaken for *psychosomatics* or it may be given a metaphysical meaning such as the relationship between body and soul. Psychophysical scaling, however, refers to the measurement of how perceived intensities vary with physical or physiological intensities. (At some meetings with psychophysicists, I have proposed the term *sensorimetrics*). The field involves many difficult problems since there is no self-evident unit of measure to use. Whereas physiologists have been spoiled in that they can always trust reliable physical units and scales, psychophysicists have had to develop their own scales based on basic mathematical principles in scaling and psychological facts concerning information processing and intersubjectivity (see part II).

Many kinds of scales have been and are still used to estimate perceptual intensities. Some are simple rating scales that do not permit any real measurements to be made; they give ratings that differ in rank order but not in distances. The most sophisticated scales, however, are the ratio scales that ambitiously provide measurements similar to physical ones, including all possible positive properties, such as an absolute zero. Still, there are also drawbacks with the so-called ratio scaling methods: They give ratings that are sufficiently valid for general descriptions of growth functions, but not for differential use and direct estimations of intensity levels (figure 3.1).

## The Borg RPE and CR10 Scales

As mentioned in chapter 1, the Borg RPE scale, a scale for ratings of perceived exertion (RPE), was developed to enable reliable and valid estimations of perceived exertion. The scale is unique because of its special use of verbal anchors to permit level determinations. The scale is also constructed so that certain psychophysical functions can be assessed according to the basic assumption that physiological strain grows linearly with exercise intensity and that perception should follow the same linear increase. This is a debatable assumption, but one that gives the scale a special metric property and makes it easy to use. It also makes it easy to compare RPE values with such physiological measurements as heart rate (HR) and oxygen consumption ($\dot{V}O_2$). The Borg RPE scale is now commonly used in exercise testing, training, and rehabilitation.

The Borg CR10 scale is similar in that it also gives reliable and valid level responses and well-defined psychophysical growth functions. The forms of these functions are, however, not determined by the form of any physiological functions or other measurements of exercise intensity, but by internal psychophysical criteria. These criteria are based on special theoretical assumptions and empirical results obtained by ratio scaling

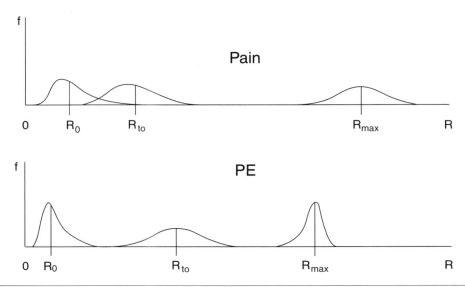

**Figure 3.1**   Hypothetical frequency distributions for pain and perceived exertion. Three fundamental distributions for each modality are drawn in the diagram. $R_0$ denotes the absolute threshold, $R_{to}$ the tolerance level, and $R_{max}$ the maximal subjective intensity. The position and range of these distributions have not been sufficiently studied scientifically. There is, however, a great need to be able to describe and understand these distributions, and other similar ones, for identification levels and adaptation levels.

methods such as ratio estimation and magnitude estimation (see chapter 4).

## When to Use the Scales

The first question often asked about using the scales is, When should people be asked to give a rating of perceived intensities? Some researchers or practitioners hesitate to use scaling because they think the methods are too unreliable, take too much time, or are not worth the effort. Some may also think that it interferes with the study they want to perform. Yet the answer to this question is simple: You can almost always use scaling, and it is often advantageous to include it in your battery of tests. Scaling can give valuable additional information for your interpretations and understanding of the subject; it does not take much time nor is it particularly problematic for the test leader nor the subject being tested. The few questions to which the subject must respond according to the scaling procedure seldom interfere with the testing process and, in fact, one can arrange the situation so that it really does not interfere. For example, the HR can be taken before the subject is asked about perceived exertion.

Throughout this book many examples are given of the use of the Borg RPE scale in labora-
tory and field situations, both scientific investigations and routine applications. The most common applications are found in exercise tests on healthy people or patients and in rehabilitation of cardiac patients. The scale is also useful to athletes for determining and monitoring the appropriate intensity level of their training. In many daily activities the scale offers an important way to compare the exertion and difficulty when using different tools, for example, how heavy or hard it is for a janitor to mop or sweep.

## What Scale to Use

Another question concerns the problem of what scale to use. This book is devoted mainly to presenting the Borg RPE scale and the Borg CR10 scale. However, the book also introduces other ratio scaling methods, such as ratio production and magnitude estimation (see chapter 4). When using magnitude estimation, people are encouraged to use numbers according to their own preferences, without any predetermined scale. The main request is that they try to use numbers in such a way that the relationship among the given numbers corresponds to the relationship among their perceived intensities.

This means that the responses concerning relationships are usable when determining relative growth functions, but not when determining any direct (*absolute*) intensity levels for certain stimuli. For example, if we just want to know how much harder a person generally perceives exercise at a work intensity (W) of 150 (150W) for 4 min than at 100W for 4 min, then magnitude estimation may be used. If we also want to know in a more absolute or "level-anchored" sense how hard these exercise intensities are perceived—for example, in relation to an individual's working capacity—then these scales cannot be used. Instead, the RPE or CR10 scales should be used because they fulfill the demands of absolute identification of levels of intensity.

The Borg RPE scale is the most commonly used scale for tests of perceived exertion. One main advantage of the RPE scale is that the given ratings grow linearly with exercise intensity, HR, and $\dot{V}O_2$. Given ratings are then easy to compare with common measurements of exercise intensity.

The Borg CR10 scale, on the other hand, is more complicated than the Borg RPE scale in its construction. It gives responses that may be said to belong to a ratio scale. The construction of the CR10 scale makes it possible to determine growth functions for different modes, to compare them with physiological growth functions, and to make direct estimates of intensity levels for interindividual comparisons. The CR10 scale is a general intensity scale that can be used to estimate most kinds of perceptual intensities. It is now commonly used to estimate pain intensity, such as angina pain or musculoskeletal pain. It is also rather commonly used in human factors and ergonomic evaluations of difficulties or complaints in manual materials handling and for other perceptions, such as taste or loudness.

A drawback of the Borg CR10 scale is that the number range, a bit smaller than that of the Borg RPE scale, is a bit too small. Also, for ratings of perceived exertion the Borg CR10 scale does not give the simple linear relationship to exercise intensity that the RPE scale does. In most situations it is preferable to use the RPE scale for perceived exertion and the CR10 scale for pain ratings. However, the CR10 scale has a wider applicability and can be used for most perceptual intensities, including perceived exertion (for more information refer to chapter 6).

# Some Misuses of the Scales to Avoid

There are some misuses of the scaling methods. A major problem is that not all people can be expected to give reliable or valid ratings according to any scaling method. A small percentage of adults, about 5% to 10% (estimates based on discussions at American College of Sports Medicine meetings), may have difficulties in understanding the instruction and the requests to respond according to the Borg RPE scale. If we include all adults in a population, including those who are far below mean intelligence and have poor verbal and mathematical abilities, the percentage may be somewhat higher. People of average intelligence or above, with a good understanding of their native language and ability to count and use numbers, should not have any difficulties using the rating scales. If difficulties arise, a complementary additional explanation should be used to correct the subjects and help them understand the procedure.

There are, however, also some errors in using the scales due to illegal copying and alterations with changes in the format, positioning of the verbal anchors, changes of adjectives and adverbs that are used as intersubjective points of reference, and alterations of the direction of intensity increase horizontally or vertically. Other violations that have been made are changes in the design, introducing colors with different emotional meaning, and so on. A very bad distortion of the CR10 scale is when the dot (•) above 10 and outside the range of numbers on the scale is changed to 10+, which simply means something more than 10. The dot means absolute maximum, and numbers higher than 10 should be possible. To avoid the "ceiling effect," there should not be a fixed endpoint. People should understand that there might be unexpectedly strong perceptions, those that are stronger than experienced before, such as "maximal pain" (e.g., an extraordinary pain during a kidney stone attack, back damage, or childbirth). Further distortions of the scales include shortening or changing the instruction. Correct instructions for the test leader and the subject are essential for administering the scale and ensuring the correct interpretation of a response.

All these changes in design, wording, spacing, and so on alter the metric properties of a scale. An expression such as "10+" is ordinal in nature and does not belong in a scale constructed to give a monotonically increasing function over the whole range of intensities, including not only low or high intensities, but also the most extreme ones, up to the strongest possible. Changing the rating scale may be a way to manipulate the responses in order to avoid more accurate or real ones. As an analogy, if the goal is to encourage people to follow the speed limits, it is not wise to end the speed scale at 70 (or 70+) mph; likewise, if the goal is to reduce obesity, it is not wise to have a weight scale end at 200 pounds.

In all cases it is of the utmost importance that the test leader who interprets a given rating understand the difficulties of scaling and use well-founded experiences and valid norms in order to arrive at the best possible interpretation. For pain ratings the subject may estimate the local intensity of an acute, burning pain or the degree of suffering in a chronic pain. If an appropriate method is not used, the subject may respond with a rating that represents more cognitive or affective components than the acute, organic, and nociceptive pain that the doctor has in mind. Thus, in many cases it is important that the test leader identify exactly the dimensions or variables to be tested and give instructions for each variable, such as the degree of local acute pain and the degree of suffering. Even with a good scaling method including instructions, valid points of reference, and so on, it is important that the test leader understand the theoretical bases of the test, has experience with the procedures, and take responsibility for the evaluations.

# PART II

# *Principles of Scaling and Using the Borg Scales*

# Chapter 4

# Psychophysical Scaling

The aim of psychophysics is to measure intensities of sensory perception and experiences such as loudness, taste, perceived exertion, and pain. The history of psychophysics dates back to the middle of the 19th century, when E.H. Weber investigated discrimination thresholds and the physicist G.T. Fechner developed methods for detection and identification (Fechner 1860). The method of limits (stimulus intensities are varied in ascending and descending series, e.g., for determination of a "just noticeable" intensity or a "just noticeable" difference) and the method of constant stimuli are still fundamental and used for the determination of *absolute thresholds* or *discrimination thresholds*. However, this book does not deal with these kinds of threshold determinations, nor with modern methods of signal-detection theory. Rather, this book deals with the scaling of perceptual intensities over a wide subjective range; please refer to Coren, Ward and Enns 1994.

Fechner (1860) presented a mathematical formula (Fechner's Law) relating the growth of sensation strength to physical intensity. According to Fechner, this relationship could best be described by a logarithmic function. Interestingly, the development of the decibel scale was based on this formula. Fechner's mathematical function did not, however, proceed from actual measures of perceptual intensities but from theoretical assumptions. The first comprehensive measurements of perceptual intensities followed the development of scaling methods such as ratio setting (halving), ratio estimation, and magnitude estimation by S.S. Stevens and his collaborators at Harvard (Stevens 1957, 1975).

Qualitative aspects of perception are difficult to assess using quantitative methods. This may

especially be true for different characteristics of pain, since it varies so much as a function of localization, time course, and emotional and cognitive factors. Sometimes a person needs to make direct comparisons of different kinds of pain, such as when comparing heart pain to pain in the stomach. It may, however, be more common to compare different kinds of perceived exertion (such as breathlessness with aches in the legs), or the difficulty of psychomotor tasks, or colors of objects in a room. For these kinds of qualities, it is rather easy to make estimations of similarity by having subjects give numerical judgments of the degree of similarity, for example, in percentages from 100% similarity (two equal objects or events) to 0 or 1% (two totally unequal objects, such as a black car and an orange). The judgment of percentage of similarity can then be analyzed by using *factor analysis,* allowing the fundamental dimensions underlying the perceptual, qualitative differences to be determined (see Eisler and Roskam 1977).

A fundamental concept in psychophysical measurement is *sameness* (or similarity) and the principle of *equal settings,* that is, the adjustment of a variable stimulus so that it is equally strong as a standard (or target) stimulus. Simple human activities have a very high level of intersubjectivity. People can rather consistently produce quantities that are equal, such as the size of a meatball, the length of a distance to a goal, the weight of a bag, and the strength of a throw (both absolute in stimulus-measures and relative, i.e., corrected according to individual strength).

This simple kind of measuring of a psychophysical event is similar to the physical operation of filling a can with sand so it is equal in weight to a certain object, except we cannot express the weight of the object as a multiple of a meaningful unit and we don't know anything directly about the weight relationship between the object and any other objects. If only equal settings are to be performed, it is impossible to scale anything. To that end, a stimulus of a given intensity (and its corresponding perception for psychophysical scaling) has to be compared with other stimuli and perceptions of different intensities so that a numerical *relationship* can be determined.

# Ratio Scaling

A simple method of scaling with a high degree of intersubjectivity (because there are no difficult mental operations involved) is *ratio setting,* such as halving or doubling. By using such simple methods, stimulus-response (S-R) relationships can be studied, and it is possible to demonstrate how sensation strength grows with physical stimulation. For example, let's start with an extremely loud sound and a treadmill exercise with a very strong perceived exertion and adjust the levels so that a test subject perceives these subjective intensities as being roughly equal. If we then let the subject adjust the loudness until it is perceived to be half as strong and slow down the speed on the treadmill until the perceived exertion feels half as strong, the resulting levels will be clearly different from the physical half values. Several such halving and doubling trials are needed at different intensity levels to obtain an S-R function. The main idea, however, is seen in figure 4.1.

Another simple example that shows how this psychophysical method of halving works is an experiment on the perception of speed when driving a car. If a person drives 50 mph and then puts the gear in neutral, letting the car slow down until the speed is perceived to be half as great, the speed will approximate 35 mph. The perception of speed grows with the square of the actual speed (Borg 1961c, 1962a). Therefore, if we perform the experiment differently, driving 50 mph and then slowing down to 25 mph, we will perceive the speed to be very much slower than half (about one fourth) of the initial speed. The perception of exertion in physical work, such as walking, shows a positively accelerating power function similar to the perception of speed (but with an exponent of about 3 [Borg 1978]; see figure 4.2 and equation (1) later in this chapter).

The direct scaling methods are called *ratio scaling methods* because they give subjective intensities on a scale that approximates a ratio scale, that is, a scale with an absolute zero and equidistant scale steps (in contrast to an interval scale, which has equal scale steps but no true zero, and in contrast to an ordinal scale, which has steps that only follow in rank order). Observe that ratio scaling in the psychophysical context involves much greater difficulties than in the physical context and cannot be expected to give perfect ratio data.

There are two main types of ratio scaling methods: the *production methods,* in which subjects produce a physical intensity corresponding to a certain subjective intensity or a fraction of a standard (e.g., ratio setting, such as halving), and the *estimation methods,* in which subjects are presented

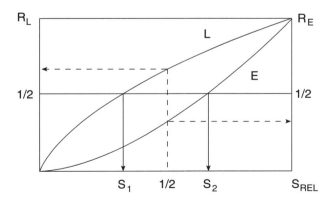

**Figure 4.1** Manner in which the perception (R) of loudness (L) and exertion (E) grows with the physical intensity (S) in a relative (REL) scale. Notice the magnitude of R when S is halved and the magnitude of S ($S_1$ and $S_2$) when R is halved.

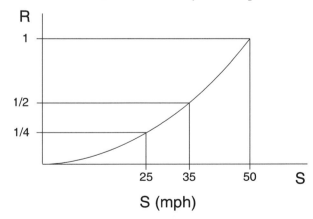

**Figure 4.2** Note how the perception of speed (R) varies with the physical speed (S) when driving a car. The variation can be described by the function $R = c \cdot S^2$ (Borg 1962a), a function similar to that for perceived exertion.

certain stimuli and are asked to try to estimate their intensities. The most common scaling method is *magnitude estimation* (ME), in which subjects respond with numbers freely and according to their own feelings, but in such a way that the relationship between the numbers corresponds to the relationship between the perceived intensities.

According to S.S. Stevens (1975), the instruction for magnitude estimation should be simple:

> The instruction may be modeled on this example: You will be presented with a series of stimuli in irregular order. Your task is to tell how intense they seem by assigning numbers to them. Call the first stimulus any number than seems appropriate to you. Then assign successive numbers in such a way that they reflect your subjective impression. There is no limit to the range of numbers that you may use. You may use whole numbers, decimals, or fractions. Try to make each number match the intensity as you perceive it.

To diminish the variance across subjects, different methods have been suggested (Borg 1977, 1982a; Zwislocki and Goodman 1980; J.C. Stevens and Marks 1980; Berglund 1991; see also Gesheider 1985).

The validity of the ratio scaling methodology is difficult to test empirically. One strong proof, in my mind, is the very high correspondence between psychophysical functions and relevant physiological ones. If we believe that most of the variation of the sensory qualities and magnitude should be possible to explain physiologically, experiments showing high psychological correlations support the validity. A unique possibility for a neurophysiological validation of the psychophysical functions for taste came up in the 1960s, when it became possible to correlate perceptual responses of taste with afferent neurological responses from the taste nerve in human beings (Borg et al. 1967). The results showed a very high psychological correspondence.

Most of the psychophysical functions obtained with ratio scaling methods may be described by simple power functions:

$$R = c \cdot S^n \tag{1}$$

where $R$ is the perceived intensity, $c$ is a measurement constant, $S$ is the physical intensity, and $n$ is the exponent that shows the appearance of the growth function (S.S. Stevens 1957, 1975). This function suggests that if the stimulus intensity is increased by a certain factor, the perceptual intensity also increases by a factor (most often another factor): "Equal $S$ ratios produce equal $R$ ratios."

However, I have modified this simple power function proposed by Stevens (Borg 1961a, 1962a) to better correspond to all kinds of psychophysical functions from different perceptual modalities and also to physiological functions, such as

---

## The Pleasure of the Unexpected: The First Neurophysical Study

Presenting results that are interesting and unexpected is something very special. This has happened to me a few times, when colleagues have remarked, "That's not possible," or maybe, "It would be fantastic if it could be done."

One of my most treasured experiences was when my colleague Professor Yngve Zottermann presented the results of our psychophysiological experiments on taste (Borg et al. 1967). Some scientists at a physiology meeting in London in 1965 talked about the possibilities of fantastic future projects in which it would be possible to compare sensory perceptions with relevant neurophysiological responses from the same human beings and not only from rats or monkeys. Yngve Zottermann, professor of physiology in Stockholm and president of the International Society of Physiological Sciences, then ran up to the floor and exclaimed: "That is just what we have done." He then gave a short presentation of our preliminary results, which showed very good correlations between perceptual and physiological response for taste perception and indicated that, to a great extent, perceptual variation could be explained physiologically. That was the first time that a psychophysical function could be traced back to a neurophysical function. It evoked great interest, and the finding is now covered in most handbooks of physiology.

Perceived exertion is a more complex modality with many physiological variables to consider—to say nothing of the psychological ones.

those showing the increase in blood lactate with increased power. Two extra constants are added to the power function, resulting in the following equation:

$$R = a + c(S - b)^n \qquad (2)$$

where $a$ and $b$ are constants that indicate the starting point of the function (or the $R_0/S_0$, i.e., the absolute threshold) or the rest value (Borg 1961a, 1962a; Mountcastle, Poggio, and Werner 1963).

## Ratio Scaling of Short-Term-Effort Perceived Exertion

In the late 1950s the new ratio scaling methods were applied to problems of perceived exertion during physical exercise. Was it possible to assess perception of exertion quantitatively and to describe its variation mathematically? Borg and Dahlström (1959, 1960) showed that such measurements could in fact be made and that perceived exertion grew according to a positively accelerated function, as did perceived speed while driving a car. That is, at a strenuous exercise intensity a small increase in physical performance is perceived as requiring a larger subjective effort than the same increase at a lower exercise intensity. In this kind of short-term performance the subjects pedaling a bicycle ergometer were asked to estimate how heavy and strenuous it felt to pedal and the degree of pedal resistance, that is, the local sensation of perceived exertion from the musculoskeletal system involved. None of the subjects had any difficulties understanding the instruction, and the test was judged to have a high degree of content validity.

The reliability of the measurements in terms of internal consistency was tested with ANOVA (analyses of variance) to estimate the proportion of the total variance that was true variance. The main formulas given by McNemar (1957) were used. However, the rules given by McNemar did not, in our case, provide an appropriate calculation of within and between variances for our sources. I therefore composed a relevant ratio by combining variances, and McNemar proposed a solution for calculating degrees of freedom (McNemar, personal communication). An intratest reliability coefficient ($r_{tt}$) was thus determined in Dahlström's and my first study, which gave $r_{tt} = .95$ in two different subexperiments and $r_{tt} = .98$ in a third experiment (Borg and Dahlström 1960).

In ratio setting (halving) the subject first has to perceive a standard intensity (such as 6 mph for 1 min) and then produce a variable intensity that is perceived to be a certain part, or ratio (e.g., half), of the standard intensity. While this is very simple and, in many modalities, convenient, it is not without its restrictions. *Time-order errors* and *adaptation effects* are but two examples of such restrictions (see S.S. Stevens 1975). These and other difficulties notwithstanding, the method has worked well with many perceptual continua. The results of the experiment by Borg and Dahlström on perceived effort and exertion during short-term work on the bicycle ergometer yielded an exponent for the psychophysical function that was slightly smaller than that for perceived speed but still above 1.0. The following equation describes the function:

$$R = a + c \cdot S^n \qquad (3)$$

where $R$ is the intensity of the perception, $a$ is a small perceptual "noise" value (about 2% to 5% of a maximal exertion) indicating a slight subjective intensity when no actual work is being performed, $c$ is the measure constant, $S$ is the physical intensity in watts, and $n$ is the exponent, which in this case is 1.6.

Subsequent studies of short-term perceived exertion for exercise on the bicycle ergometer using other psychophysical methods have also

---

## *Another Pleasure of the Unexpected: The Generic Power Function*

When I gave my first introductory talk about perceived exertion in Pittsburgh in 1967, I presented my general psychophysical equation with two extra constants, $R = a + c(S - b)^n$. One psychology professor, an expert in psychophysics, told me that this was not a new idea since Mountcastle (a famous physiologist) had already presented this equation in 1963. I was happy to inform him that I had presented the same equation in 1961.

yielded exponents of about 1.6 (Borg 1962a; Borg, Edström, and Marklund 1970). In this form of heavy ergometer exercise the ratio scaling methods give reliable results in the form of highly replicable growth functions.

Experiments on subjective force of hand grip while squeezing a dynamometer have given exponents of about 1.7 (J.C. Stevens and Mach 1959), and experiments on subjective foot pressure 1.6 (Eisler 1962). Other experiments on muscular activities, including subjective heaviness in weight lifting, have also shown exponents above 1.0 (see S.S. Stevens 1975). The high similarity among obtained exponents for different kinds of muscular work is an important validation of the methods with regard to growth functions. Exponents for other sensory modalities are of a different size, some being clearly below 1.0 (brightness 0.2 to 0.4, and loudness 0.4 to 0.7) and others much above 1.0 (perceived electric stimulation around 3.0, and perceived exertion in walking also around 3.0). These exponents are founded on group functions for competent observers. When we analyze individual differences, however, we do not find the desired and necessary validity (S.S. Stevens 1975). For differential use and predictions of individual differences, the ratio scaling methods do not work well. To improve the validity by using physiological criteria or performance criteria, other methods, such as Borg's rating methods, must be used.

## Ratio Scaling of Long-Term-Effort Perceived Exertion

Several minutes of heavy work involving large muscle groups puts a great strain on the cardiopulmonary system. Thus, demands on the individual are, in part, different from those during short-term work, especially work of just a few seconds, in which peripheral sensations in the skin, muscles, and joints dominate. During work of longer duration, the load may give rise to many sensations, both peripheral and "central," and sometimes also to special symptoms of clinical diagnostic value. Perceived exertion during such exercise has been studied in many experiments using different methods (see also chapter 8). All psychophysical experiments have given positively accelerating functions with exponents around 1.6 (Borg 1961b, 1962a, 1972; Noble et al. 1983; Borg, Ljunggren, and Ceci 1985).

During treadmill tests, when the individual has to walk or run, usually under conditions of stepwise increases in speed or slope, the physical strain and the perception of exertion is rather similar to exercise on a bicycle ergometer. In one experiment a group of males had to walk at zero grade for 4 min at several different speeds from 1 to 6 mph. The following power function was obtained:

$$R = 1 + 0.066(S - 1)^3 \qquad (4)$$

where $R$ is the intensity of perceived exertion, the first number 1 denotes the value of the perceptual noise level (which is equal to the $R$ value arbitrarily set at 1 for $S = 1$ mph), 0.066 is the measure constant, $S$ is the physical speed in miles per hour, the second number 1 shows the starting point of the curve in miles per hour, and 3 is the exponent (Borg 1973b; see figure 4.3).

In this group of rather fit subjects (split into two groups), perceived exertion increased only slightly when speed was increased from 0 to 3 mph. After that point, however, the intensity of the perception increased greatly. Individual differences are, of course, large, and for less-fit subjects perceived exertion will start to increase much earlier. The growth function is rather similar to that for blood lactate.

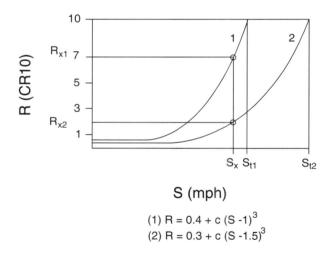

(1) $R = 0.4 + c (S - 1)^3$
(2) $R = 0.3 + c (S - 1.5)^3$

**Figure 4.3** The figure shows how perceived exertion (R) increases with speed (S) in walking. The two curves represent two subjects, one (2) with a good walking capacity (maximum speed $S_{t2}$) and the other (1) with a capacity that is 75% of subject 2's capacity (maximum speed $S_{t1}$). The perceived exertion at a submaximal level ($S_x$) is perceived to be 3.5 times higher by subject 1 ($R_{x1}$) than by subject 2 ($R_{x2}$).

The common ratio scaling methods (e.g., ME) were found to work well and, for short-term exercise, give reliable results in the form of reproducible growth functions. The validity of the methods with regard to individual functions and levels of perceived exertion for different workloads, however, is not satisfactory. Mainly nonsignificant correlations are found between ratings and HR. This is because ME methods instruct people to use any numbers they choose according to their own feelings and conceptions of numbers without any restrictions to a common response scale (S.S. Stevens 1971). One person may therefore use a rather high number, such as 40, for a first weak intensity, while another person uses only 10. The main concern is not what number the subjects use, but how they relate the perceptions and numbers to each other. If two subjects are given a second workload that both perceive to be twice as heavy, the first subject should rate it 80 and the second 20. In order for a ratio scaling method to be valid for interindividual comparisons of intensity levels, some restrictions and anchors of intersubjective relevance must be inferred.

## Ratio Scaling of Pain

In this book, qualitative aspects of pain are dealt with only roughly, since the methodological problems presented here concern degrees of magnitude within certain dimensions. It is, however, also possible to use some quantitative methods to determine qualities and fundamental dimensions. The different qualities are commonly taken more or less for granted as a starting point. If there is a need to quantify different qualities, such as the sensory component and the affective component in studies of pain, these have to be assessed separately, for example, as was done by Swedborg, Borg, and Sarnelid (1981).

Scaling experimental pain has been done in a number of studies (see Price 1988; Turk and Melzack 1992) using healthy subjects as well as patients. Linearly or positively accelerating functions have been obtained with ratio scaling methods, for example, for dental pain and somatosensory perception of pressure, cold, contact, and heat-induced pain.

A fundamental contribution to the research on pain using ratio scaling methods has been done by Gracely and his collaborators (Gracely 1979) and Rollman (1977). Gracely compared different scaling techniques including cross-modal match-

ing (CMM). When using CMM, the magnitude of pain is compared with the magnitude of another sensory perception. The subject may thus be asked to adjust the intensity of force of hand grip or loudness to his or her perception of pain. Since the psychophysical functions of these other modalities are known, a measure of pain may be obtained. Number production (as in ME) may also be considered a kind of CMM. In an attempt to improve the scaling methods, Gracely also studied verbal descriptors in order to locate their position on a ratio scale (Gracely et al. 1978; cf. Borg 1973a, 1982a). For clinical use Gracely has developed a multistage procedure according to which the patient first has to respond to a series of experimental pain stimuli (using, for example, the Visual Analog Scale [VAS], defined a little later), then match experimental pain to his or her clinical pain, and finally estimate the clinical pain using the first response scale. Interesting results have been obtained with this procedure (Gracely 1979; Price et al. 1983), but the technique is time-consuming and not as easily used as one simple response scale.

In one of the latest studies on pain using ME, Algom and Lubel (1994) compared the perception of labor pain with memories of the same pain. As the measurement of the pain-inducing stimuli, the peak intensity (pressure) of uterine contractions was determined by tocography (a physiological method giving objective measurements of the strength and course of contractions). Rather large variations were obtained among subjects, showing both positively and negatively accelerated functions. The mean functions were, however, positively accelerating with an exponent of about 1.4 for the perception of pain and with somewhat higher exponents for the memory of pain. Unfortunately, the method used did not permit valid individual differences of levels of intensity to be studied.

The most commonly used scale is the Visual Analog Scale (VAS), which consists of a line, often 10 cm long, the endpoints of which often are denoted "minimal" and "maximal" (or, instead of "maximal," "most intense pain imaginable"); the individual is instructed to make a mark indicating the magnitude of the perception (Price 1994). The VAS is not as good a ratio scaling method as, for example, ME (see Neely 1995), but it may be used as such a scale in some situations, especially at low to rather high submaximal intensities. The psychophysical functions may then be described by power functions, and exponents equal to or greater than 1.0 have been obtained. The size of the exponent is still debatable, since the absolute starting point of the function is difficult to assess and the value of this point influences the exponent quite a bit. This does not matter a great deal when studying individual differences in intensity levels, however, since the reliability of VAS responses has been shown to be high over a wide range of suprathreshold intensities (see Price 1994).

Another common, reliable method is Finger Span. Using this method, the subject is asked to adjust the span between the thumb and the index finger (or the middle finger) to indicate the degree of pain. This method has been used to study dental pain (Franzén and Ahlquist 1989) and is especially useful in situations in which the subject must respond quickly and is unable to use words or numbers.

## Interindividual and Other Interprocess Comparisons

To understand and appreciate the difficulties in scaling, we have to consider the different factors and comparisons involved when a person gives a certain response in a specific situation. When we want to study the effect of a given stimulation, such as a certain workload, on perceived exertion or a new pain therapy, we often want to focus on a specific sensory perception and its changes over time and in context. To be sure that we are making the correct observations, we must control many influencing factors and specify the comparisons we want to make.

Assessments of intensities always involve many different kinds of comparisons. We may want to make rather simple comparisons of intensities within a certain modality, for example, subjective weight or perceived exertion for one or a few subjects. As an example of a more complicated comparison, when testing athletes on the bicycle ergometer, we may find that the leg exertion of the runner is greater than the breathlessness of the cyclist. Sometimes we need to make very complex interprocess comparisons involving different modalities, different individuals, and variables from different disciplines (perceptual, physiological, and behavioral).

How can we measure something as subjective as human perception? Subjective symptoms are uncertain and private. By developing reliable scaling methods with precise instructions, we find that the quantification of subjective symptoms is well justified. The validity of the scaling methods can be proven using physiological correlates with subsequent prediction of behavior and physical performances.

The first thing we often want to identify is the modality in question and the specific quality of interest within that modality, for example, the modality of overall perceived exertion and the specific quality of breathlessness, or the modality of taste and the quality of bitterness. These sensory perceptions do not exist in an empty or neutral sphere, but in a mental context of memo-

---

## The Problem of Interpersonal Comparisons

Problems of subjectivity, interindividual comparisons, and the units used in scaling are long-standing philosophical issues in the theory of knowledge. One individual does not have certain knowledge of another person's perception. We can never creep under the skin of another person and see with her eyes, hear with her ears, or feel with her skin. For example, does person A perceive the color red in the same way as person B? Does person A have the same conscious mental experience as person B? Does person A's description of a great ache in the legs or a strong feeling of breathlessness have the same meaning as that of person B?

There is a need to clarify these concepts both from an epistemological point of view and to enhance human communication. We need a working theory concerning subjectivity to help us develop methods to quantify subjective symptoms and make reliable, valid intensity determinations and interpersonal comparisons. Quine, a famous modern philosopher, notes the importance of "shared stimulus meaning," that is, fundamental intersubjective agreement about the meaning of objects and events. He states that "the requirement of intersubjectivity is what makes science objective" (Quine 1990).

## My Perceived Exertion Is Less Than Your Heart Rate

Perceptions are subjective phenomena, unsure and private, and difficult to measure. We make many difficult subjective comparisons daily without much hesitation. We sometimes use analogies when we want to express the magnitude of a sensation, for example, by the distance between hands ("I love you *this* much"), by drawing a line, or by using concepts from other modalities, such as the sourness of a lemon or the sound of an ambulance. It is interesting to note how fundamental interprocess comparisons form our experiences and emotions and affect everyday communication. Consider Shakespeare's verse in *A Midsummer Night's Dream:* "Your threats have no more strength than her weak prayers." In this verse Shakespeare makes three different kinds of subjective comparisons: interindividual, interevent (intermodal), and intermagnitude (ordinary strength to weak). The following statements illustrate similar interprocess comparisons: "Today you have to look after the kids because my training is more important than your visit with your parents," or "Your goal-shot accuracy isn't worth half of Bill's quickness."

ries, ideas, and emotions interacting with other perceptions in a special network. The purpose of a study may also concern intermodal comparisons, for example, between the taste, smell, color, and temperature of a wine, or between the physical effort and mental difficulty of a psychomotor task.

When making these comparisons we often want to study different intensity levels over a wide range, from minimal to maximal. All these simultaneous processes have a certain duration or a specific time course that further complicates things. To this we can add the physical extension over the body and the situation of our activities, both the physical and the psychosocial. There are also many different kinds of person-by-situation interactions, meaning that similar stimuli may provoke different responses, depending on the specific situation in question. One last thing to consider is the interdisciplinary factor, especially for simultaneous determinations of psychological and physiological processes.

The problem of interindividual comparisons should be emphasized. When thinking of all these factors and interacting variables, we may despair about the possibility of assessing one person's sensory perception and comparing it with another's. Remember that a perception is always subjective in that it is private and not directly assessable via performance or physiological responses. The problem is not made easier by the fact that there are many different methods involved, each revealing different aspects of perception and each fraught with different sources of error. No single method exists that can be used to measure all variables and that facilitates all interprocess comparisons. Many of these interprocess comparisons may be classified into four categories (in a four-squared table): those that concern *relationships*, those that concern *levels,* those that concern *intraindividual* (or general) processes, and those that concern *interindividual* (differential) ones.

## Relationships and Levels

The ratio scaling methods are very well suited for determining S-R functions describing *relative* growth curves. Such functions give important information about general relationships between intensities, but not about any "absolute" or direct intensity levels. They are similar to measurements in physics, in which an arbitrary and reliable but "meaningless" unit is chosen.

If a competent observer states that a certain stone is half as big as another stone, most people may agree; that is, there is a high degree of interindividual agreement about the relationship. This invariance of relationship supports the idea of intersubjectivity—good agreement among people. If, however, the observer claims that a certain stone, which is as big as a football, is small, some people may not agree, especially not a small child.

The fact that psychophysical ratio scaling methods provide only relationships between stimuli is a great drawback that still is not fully recognized in psychology. A further example: A certain weight, although two times heavier than a standard weight, is not necessarily "heavy." Indeed, a trained weight lifter and a child may perceive the *relationship* between two weights to be the same, but the "absolute" exertion in lifting them will be higher for the child. In this example, there is no *unit* that is anchored in such a way that it can be said that intensity A is weak but intensity B is strong. We can only say that B is *x* times stronger than A, but we cannot make any "absolute" determinations of intensity levels.

One special problem with Stevens's ratio scaling methods is that the variation between individual exponents is rather large. Differences between modalities are well established and significant, with exponents varying from about 0.3 for perceived brightness to about 3.0 for perceived exertion in walking (and perceived electric stimulation). But intraindividual fluctuation is also substantial (20% or more), and interindividual variation even greater (e.g., exponent variation from 0.9 to 2.5 for perceived exertion in bicycling, with a median value of 1.6 [Borg 1962a, 1972]). Corresponding determinations with my scaling methods result in much less variability.

The great individual variation among exponents is most often not a meaningful indicator of differences in sensory functioning, but rather of differences in rating behavior (Borg and Borg 1992). Stevens's opinion was that the individual exponents should not be taken literally. Since the functional characteristics of the human sensory system are essentially the same in most subjects (except in pathological cases), the differences found between subjects should depend primarily on differences in rating behavior (response bias). Averaging data that are obtained from many individuals using both estimation and production methods should give the most valid psychophysical functions with exponents that are representative of fundamental sensory processes and physiologically based transductional differences between modalities.

Great individual variability is, of course, rather disappointing and leaves us with only crude measures for individual comparisons of *relative* growth functions. What then about the intensity *levels?* Levels are the other, and more difficult, part of intersubjectivity. Remember the statement by Quine (1990) that intersubjectivity is fundamental to objectivity. Quine (1987) also states, however:

> There is no place in science for bigness, because of this lack of boundary: but there is a place for the relation of biggerness. Here we see the familiar and widely applicable rectification of vagueness: disclaim the vague positive and cleave to the precise comparative.

Quine's statement concerns the physical sciences. A biological system, however, has its boundaries from rest, or minimum, to a maximum level, and intensity variation is possible within these limits. Thus, according to my range model, something is big or small depending on its position in the range.

## Ratio Scaling of Relationships, Not of Levels

Stevens and Ekman were both very negative toward simple rating methods and never fully understood one of the main problems with ratio scaling regarding "level determinations." Stevens wanted to use methods that were as close as possible to those used in natural science, where arbitrary and "meaningless" units are used. A drawback with the ratio scaling method, however, is that people use numbers as a personal secondary "modality" and not as abstract, mathematical concepts. When I tested lumber workers from the northern part of Sweden in 1960, I explained the ratio estimation method in which one perception of a stimulus is called "100" and a weaker one should be estimated in relation to this. If the weaker is half as strong, the subject should say "50"; if it is only 10% as strong, the subject should say "10," and so forth. Trying to explain the method simply, I used an example with a coin and said: "If you have one krona (or one dollar) and one 25-öring (a quarter), what percent is the 25-öring of the krona?" Most people answered 25, but some gave other answers, such as 4. To avoid the difficulties with percentage estimates and at the same time facilitate direct estimations of levels of intensity, a special category-rating scale was developed that later became the Borg RPE scale.

# Interindividual and Intraindividual Concerns

I proposed the *range model* (Borg 1961a, 1962a, 1990) as a working model permitting interindividual comparisons of perceived exertion. A main assumption of this model is that perceptual intensities are approximately equal for different people at each individual's subjective maximal exertion. This is true in spite of the fact that the stimulus intensities at this maximum may differ. The range from zero (or an extremely small intensity at threshold or at rest) to the maximal intensity is used as a frame of reference. The intensity of a perception is thus determined by its position in the range (see figure 4.4). In the field of perceived exertion the assumption of similarity at maximal intensity may be validated against the maximum in physiological responses, such as HR and blood lactate.

The model can also be used to make relative evaluations of different physiological measurements. In the case of linear relationships, as with HR/power output functions, the range model can be used in a simple way as predicted by the Karvonen equation (Karvonen, Kentala, and Musta 1957). According to this equation, the relative intensity of a response ($RR_x$) is the increase above rest calculated as a percentage of the range from rest to maximum. In some other cases the exponent should also be taken into consideration (see equations (6) and (7) for relative response [$RR$] and relative stimulus [$RS$] intensities).

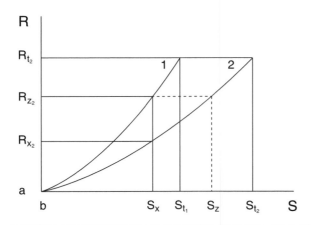

**Figure 4.4** The psychophysical functions for two subjects (1 and 2). S is the physical intensity (e.g., weight in kilograms), R is the perceptual intensity, and $R_t$ is the terminal subjective intensity (e.g., the heaviest weight a person can lift), which is set equal for both subjects according to the range theory.

Obtaining individual measurements of $c$ is a problem for interindividual comparisons. According to the model, $c$ in the general equation (2) is solved thus:

$$c = \frac{R_t - a}{(S_t - b)^n} \times 100 \qquad (5)$$

where $R_t$ and $S_t$ stand for terminal (maximal) values for the response ($R$) and for the stimulus ($S$). The fraction is then multiplied by 100 to avoid decimals. The constants $a$ and $b$ show the starting point of the curve. For physiological variables, $a$ is usually positive (e.g., a rest value of 1 mmol of blood lactate), and $b$ is sometimes positive (e.g., 50 W on the ergometer before the lactate starts to increase). For perceptual variables, $a$ and $b$ are most often zero, except in the case of perception of exertion; in this case, $a$ is often a small percentage of the maximal exertion, but $b$ is usually zero (except for perceived exertion in walking, where it may approximate 1 mph). The constant $a$ is the value at which there is not yet a response to $S$ (the value at rest), and the range $R_t - a$ is the range (frame of reference) for interprocess comparisons. The relative intensity of a response may be calculated directly or by inserting the expression for $c$ in equation (2) and multiplying it by 100:

$$RR_x = \left( \frac{S_x - b}{S_t - b} \right)^n \times 100 \qquad (6)$$

As an example of an application of equation (6), imagine that you are going to take a brisk walk and want to know the perceived exertion for a walk of half an hour. You know that if you exert yourself to the maximum, you can walk 2.5 miles during half an hour (a speed of 5 mph). According to equation (4), the exponent is 3 and the $b$ value is 1 mph (at 1 mph there is no real exertion). If you walk at 4 mph, the relative response in percentage of maximum is $RR_x = [(4 - 1)/(5 - 1)]^3 \times 100 = 42\%$. The high exponent means that perceived exertion is very sensitive to changes in speed. If you walk at 3.5 mph, the percentage will be 24%, and if your speed is 4.5 mph, it will be 67%.

If we want to calculate a relative stimulus intensity, as we might in order to predict an effective therapy from some physiological measurements, we can start from response measurements. We can use the human being as a measuring instrument, as is done in psychometric determinations of the difficulty of test items, and determine the intensity of the stimulus. This relative stimulus intensity (*RS*) may then be calculated in the same way as in the preceding example, but using response measurements:

$$RS_x = \left( \frac{R_x - a}{R_t - a} \right)^{1/n} \times 100 \qquad (7)$$

To illustrate the application of equation (7), we may use the same example as before. Assume that you can walk with a maximal speed of 5 mph, and you want to know the time you should spend walking 2 miles in order to exert yourself to 40% of maximal perceived exertion. We can insert 40 into the equation, and if we neglect the *a* value (since it is so small and amounts to only one or a few percent of maximum), we get $RS_x = (40/100)^{1/3} \times 100 = 73.7\%$. This means a walking speed of 3.7 mph (73.7% of maximal speed of 5 mph), in other words 2 miles in about half an hour (33 minutes to be more exact).

Support for the range model is obtained from general theoretical ideas, common sense derived from daily living experiences, and anecdotal evidence from psychology. From the preceding examples, insight about how the range model works in individual cases is also obtained. The major problem is, however, how the model can be defended and how it works interindividually. In psychophysics the new model was not appreciated by leading psychophysicists, such as Ekman, Parducci, and Stevens (personal communication). Also, from a purely philosophical point of view, the assumption of the "sameness" (or very high similarity) of perceptual intensities at maximal performances may be judged to be invalid since it is not empirically possible to verify or falsify it in an absolute sense.

A more practical argument against the idea of sameness comes from the observations (made by Parducci) that an athlete, such as a racing cyclist, can exert himself or herself to a much greater degree than an ordinary person and will, at his or her maximal performance, most likely feel a higher degree of perceived exertion. Thus, it was argued that a model assuming sameness must be false.

It is certainly true that during an extreme performance an athlete may, in general, experience a more intense perception of exertion than a less-motivated person. However, that does not invalidate the model. We must start with an assumption of sameness, that people perceive the world in approximately the same way and that when they perform to their maximum they experience similar sensations. To me this assumption has an epistemic priority; the fact that people differ from each other can be understood only as a deviation from something that is similar. In a group of subjects, one person's deviation, indicating dissimilarity, is a deviation from a mean value, indicating similarity. And similarity is difficult to understand if we cannot accept the idea of sameness. This does not mean absolute sameness in perceptions. I cannot have the same perception as another person, but I can identify the same objects or events, and I can perceive the same relationships, both relatively (events to each other) and absolutely (relative to my maximum as an internal point of reference).

## *Special Examples of the Range Model?*

After I had presented my range model during a seminar, one of my doctoral students spontaneously interposed: "This must be the same idea that my father used to refer to when our family went hiking. When my older brothers wanted me to carry as much as they did, my father used to say, 'Everyone according to his or her ability.'"

When I discussed this 10 years ago with my then 25-year-old daughter (who has a much better knowledge of the Bible than I have), she immediately responded by saying that the model fits very well with the text in the Bible when Jesus talks about the widow's last farthing:

And he looked up and saw the rich men that were casting their gifts into the treasury. And he saw a certain poor widow casting in thither two mites. And he said, "Of a truth, I say unto you, this poor widow cast in more than they all: for all these did of their superfluity cast in unto the gifts; but she of her want did cast in all the living that she had." (Luke 21:1-4, American Standard Bible 1901)

# Chapter 5

# The Borg RPE Scale

The common Borg RPE scale (from ratings of perceived exertion [RPE] that I constructed; see Borg 1970b) has become popular because it has some special properties and is easy to understand and use. Other scales, such as ratio scales, have also been applied to estimate RPE. However, the ratio scales do not function well for direct level estimates or interindividual comparisons, and the ordinary rating scales (e.g., symmetrical scales with steps from 1 to 7) are less valid and have a rather bad reputation among psychophysicists.

When scaling perceived exertion, we want to know not only how much heavier one exercise is than another one, but also if it is heavy or not. We want to tell a person—for example, a patient after a cardiac infarction—that he or she should exercise at a moderate intensity. We want to be able to communicate about intensity levels in a way that is relevant for each individual. We then have to build upon each person's own inner frame of reference and use a language consisting of ordinary, simple expressions denoting grades of intensity, anchored individually, but chosen so as still to give a high degree of intersubjective agreement.

In spite of the condemnation of category scaling by both Stevens and Ekman (and most experts in scaling), we started to use some simple rating methods in connection with physical stress tests on bicycle ergometers in Umeå, Sweden. The first scale was a simple symmetrical 7-grade rating scale with all numbers anchored with simple verbal expressions (1-very, very, light through 7-very, very hard). We thus followed the old tradition in psychometrics reported by Guilford (1954). Rather high correlations were obtained between given ratings and simultaneously registered heart rate (HR). However, since some subjects during an exercise test with stepwise increased workloads had to exercise at many different loads, for example, at five to seven different loads, we wanted the subjects to have different categories and numbers from which to select at each successive load.

We then increased the numbers of the scale till we had a 21-grade scale (1-21). This scale gave very high correlations with HR (around $r_{xy} = .85$, higher than the 7-grade scale), while Stevens's ratio scaling methods gave no or very low correlations. This 21-grade scale was used for several years during the 1960s in Sweden. However, as reported by Borg (1962a, 1970b), there was a drawback with the scale. It gave neither responses growing according to the positively accelerating functions obtained by the ratio scaling methods nor the linear increase that should agree with the physiological energy demands. The obtained ratings instead followed a slightly negatively accelerated function with exercise intensity and HR (see Borg 1962b).

## Construction of the Scale

The Borg RPE scale was constructed from the knowledge gained from our psychophysical and physiological experiments. The results from the 21-grade rating scale were of special interest. On that scale, 17 corresponded roughly to a HR of 170 beats per minute (bpm) in a normal, healthy group of middle-aged men and women exercising on a bicycle ergometer with stepwise increased loads every sixth minute. Since in healthy persons 170 bpm was a common point of reference in estimating submaximal measurements of working capacity, the rating 17 was easy to compare with the HR divided by 10.

However, since there was a nonlinear relation between ratings and workloads, interpolations and extrapolations in the HR-rating and rating-workload diagrams were somewhat difficult to make. To overcome this difficulty, make the ratings grow linearly with workload, and at the same time simplify comparisons between ratings and HR over a wide range of intensities, I changed the scale by replacing the verbal anchors and straightening the curve down to a rest value (or a perceptual noise level close to rest). I did this by plotting the 21-grade scale to workload and HR and then replacing and moving down some expressions to correspond to a linear growth function (see figure 5.1).

I chose the number 6 as the starting point, since a low resting HR estimate for many adults is close to 60 (60 = 10 × 6). Every uneven number was verbally anchored as seen in figure 5.2. Starting with 6 (instead of zero) shows that the scale is not a ratio scale with an absolute zero. The RPE scale was also constructed to give a fairly linear increase with HR (and $\dot{V}O_2$) during cycling (and later also during running).

I gave the first presentation of the scale at a seminar for clinical physiology in Sweden in 1966; hospitals in Scandinavia, and after 1967 in the United States, began to use it during stress tests. To improve the precision of the verbal anchors and the linearity of the scale to further facilitate interpolations, I made a minor change to the scale in the 1980s (Borg 1985). Number 6 was anchored with the expression "No exertion at all,"

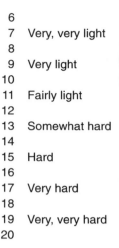

| 6 | |
| 7 | Very, very light |
| 8 | |
| 9 | Very light |
| 10 | |
| 11 | Fairly light |
| 12 | |
| 13 | Somewhat hard |
| 14 | |
| 15 | Hard |
| 16 | |
| 17 | Very hard |
| 18 | |
| 19 | Very, very hard |
| 20 | |

**Figure 5.2**   The old RPE scale.

and the expression at number 7 was moved up half a step. "Very, very" was changed to the slightly stronger and more precise "Extremely" and "Fairly light" to "Light." Number 20 was anchored with the expression "Maximal exertion" (see figure 5.3).

These changes were based on a combination of available material and a special study by Borg and Lindblad (1976) on the interpretation and precision of 37 different verbal anchors from "Minimum" to "Almost maximal." In the study, groups of subjects rated the conceived intensities behind the expressions. Interpretation and precision were defined operationally by the results from the study. Interpretation was defined by the mean (and median) position on the scale, and precision by the relative dispersion around the mean (see also Borg 1964).

Number 20 on the scale refers to a kind of "absolute maximum," an intensity that most people never will have reached previously in their lives. It is thus a kind of hypothetical construct. According to the definition and instruction, 19 should be the highest intensity that most people have ever experienced in running extremely hard for several minutes or carrying objects that are so heavy that they can hardly manage to perform the task. Most people, however, may be able to imagine an intensity that is still somewhat stronger (see instructions to the scale in chapter 7 and the appendix). The construction of the RPE scale is unique, and the scale may be considered an equidistant interval scale. The final RPE scale is shown in figure 5.3 (Borg 1985, 1994a).

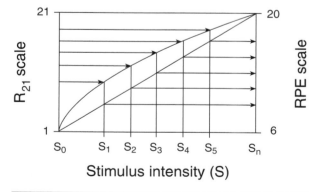

**Figure 5.1**   The theoretical principle behind the change of the symmetrical 21-grade ($R_{21}$) scale to the special, "linear" RPE scale.

| | |
|---|---|
| 6 | No exertion at all |
| 7 | |
| 8 | Extremely light |
| 9 | Very light |
| 10 | |
| 11 | Light |
| 12 | |
| 13 | Somewhat hard |
| 14 | |
| 15 | Hard   (heavy) |
| 16 | |
| 17 | Very hard |
| 18 | |
| 19 | Extremely hard |
| 20 | Maximal exertion |

Borg RPE scale
© Gunnar Borg, 1970, 1985, 1994, 1998

**Figure 5.3**   The Borg RPE scale, the 15-grade scale for ratings of perceived exertion (RPE).

# Reliability of the Scale

The reliability of subjective ratings is often questioned since subjectivity implies something not only private but often also uncertain (see chapter 4). If the attribute to be estimated is something rather vague with a small range of variation or if bad instruction is given, the reliability will often be low. A rather obscure trait, a vague feeling or attitude, is difficult to measure, and few grades (three to five) should be used. The perception of exertion is, however, a very concrete experience that is easy to describe and identify over a large range of intensities. It is as distinct a perception as the sourness of a fruit or the color of a flower. It also has many physiological cues that might help the subject to identify a certain intensity level.

The reliability of ratings of perceived exertion has been found to be high in many investigations using different kinds of procedures. The basic definition of reliability is the proportion of the total variance that is true variance (that is, the internal consistency); it is therefore desirable to determine reliability from intratest correlations and from ANOVA. The reproducibility of repeated measurements is then considered broadly, allowing room for repetitions within a test session or by using alternative forms in the experimental design. Retest correlations are also very informative, as are indirect reliability estimates from validity coefficients.

Previous experiments with ratio scaling resulted in reliability coefficients much above .90 (Borg 1962a), leading to the prediction that it should be possible to obtain high reliability coefficients with measurements from the new RPE scale. The first category scale with numbers from 1 to 21 had also given high reliability and validity coefficients, and the change from 21 steps to 16 on the new scale was not expected to affect the reliability (Guilford 1954), especially since the new RPE scale with 16 steps improved the linearity with power level and HR.

By the end of the 1960s there was enough theoretical evidence and conclusions from some pilot studies regarding both the reliability and validity of the new RPE scale to warrant an official presentation and publication of the scale (Borg 1970b). Many studies have since been performed analyzing the reliability in different situations and using different approaches for estimations. In this chapter, I present a selection of representative studies.

## Parallel Test Reliability

Correlations obtained from calculations based on two different parallel scales are one way to estimate reliability. Since the RPE scale is constructed mainly to give measurements of exercise intensity, HR may be regarded as a parallel test. Very high correlations (reliability coefficients above .90) have been obtained between RPE and HR.

In a study by Borg (1972), subjects rated perceived exertion on the RPE scale and by using a method in which they had to estimate the exertion as a percentage of a conceived maximal exertion. For exercise on a bicycle ergometer the correlation at 100 W (workload) between RPE values and percentage ratings was .70. At 150 W the corresponding correlation was .87. These are surprisingly high correlations since they refer to only one level of physical intensity. When reliability is estimated in ordinary psychometric performance tests of difficulty, a large range of intensities (items of different difficulty) is used rather than only one intensity level (items of equal difficulty). When responses from the whole test with items of different difficulty are obtained, correlations above .90 may be predicted.

I also estimated reliability coefficients using a different psychophysical method (Borg 1974a). Subjects were instructed to make estimates of exertion in relation to a very special anchor: their notion of a maximal subjective intensity of sourness, which was called "100." HR and RPE values were registered simultaneously for several minutes' exercise on the bicycle ergometer. High correlation coefficients were obtained for the different workloads, ranging from .50 to .70 for 150 and 200 W. For the total work test the correlation between percentage ratings and RPE was .94.

In a study on the reliability and validity of four different rating scales (Borg 1973c), two groups of 18- to 19-year-old male military Swedish conscripts exercised on the bicycle ergometer several minutes according to two different test protocols. Two scales were used by each subject, and HR was also registered. The RPE scale (method *a*) was compared with ratings using an 11-cm horizontal line (method *b*), to the left of which was written "no exertion at all" and to the right "maximal exertion." The other two scales were the old 21-grade scale (method *c*) and a 9-point graded scale (method *d*) designed in Pittsburgh by Noble, Robertson, and MacBurney (personal communication). There were 132 subjects in the first work test, divided in two groups. One group had to rate exertion using methods *a* and *b*, and the other group used methods *c* and *d*. The correlation between the RPE scale (*a*) and the line scale (*b*) was .93 and between the old 21-grade scale (*c*) and the 9-grade scale (*d*) .92. In a second experiment 89 subjects participated in a similar scale comparison, but using a different test protocol. Correlation coefficients of similar magnitude were obtained.

## Intratest Reliability

A drawback of parallel testing is that subjects may know that they are exercising at the same workloads. Even if there is a brief time between the ratings using the different scales, subjects may know that the perceived exertion should be about the same. It is thus only the similarities of the response scale and their constraints that are tested. In the intratest correlational analyses previously described for short-duration exercises (which used ratio scaling methods and had reliability coefficients clearly above .90 [Borg and Dahlström 1960]), it was possible to get several responses for the same workloads by mixing and randomizing the workload presentations over a period of time. The fatigue effects for such short-term work are not as great as they are for long-term exercise of a steady-state character. For the latter kind of exercise it is difficult to get good intratest

reliability estimations since the test has to be spread over time with several trials on different days to avoid fatigue effects or memories of previously given ratings for identified workloads.

One way to avoid these difficulties is to make a calculation analogous to the split-half technique used in many psychometric studies of mental abilities. If a test with several items is divided in two halves, for example, by picking all odd items in one half and all even items in another half, and the results combined within each half, two estimates can be obtained for each individual, and the correlation between these estimates should reveal the degree of reliability.

In an exercise test with several workloads, RPE values from all loads can be plotted for each individual. Instead of directly comparing the different ratings, it is then possible to calculate one value from the odd data points and one from the even data points. With at least four points in the diagram, the workload for a certain reference level in RPE can then be calculated so that two estimates can be determined for the same test and compared. The result can most easily be expressed in two measurements at the workload (W) for a certain reference level, for example, RPE 15 giving $W_{R15(1)}$ and $W_{15(2)}$. This method was used in a study by Borg, Herbert, and Ceci (1984) for running at different speeds. A reliability coefficient of .93 was obtained.

## Retest Reliability

Retest reliability coefficients have been obtained from several studies in running. In one test by Borg and Ohlsson (1975) subjects had to run 800 m three times at three different speeds according to a certain instruction. HR and RPE values were collected after each run. The correlations between HR from the first and second run was .74, from the first and third run .64, and from the second and the third run .89. The corresponding correlations between RPE values were .75, .69, and .87. The subjects also had to run 1,200 m at two different speeds. The correlation between HR from the first and second run was .87 and for the RPE values from the first and second run .91. All correlations showed that the retest reliability was very satisfactory and as good for RPE values as for HR.

In a study by Ceci and Hassmén (1991) results from running on a treadmill were compared with running on an outdoor track on two different occasions at certain RPE levels. High test-retest reliability was found for both situations and sessions. Correlation coefficients on RPE data for both velocity and HR levels were .90 or higher.

In a study by Komi and Karppi (1977) a sample of 14 male and 22 female twin pairs was tested on the bicycle ergometer with increasing loads. RPE data were collected together with HR. The subjects were tested two times with one week of rest between, after a first maximum test. Each pair was tested simultaneously, and to prevent the subjects from communicating with each other, they gave the ratings silently by making a mark on a line beside which the expressions from the RPE scale were written. In the second and third test the loads were chosen to correspond to 35%, 50%, 70%, 90%, and 100% of each person's maximal capacity. The retest correlation of the responses from the lightest work (35% of maximum) was low, $r_{tt} = .37$. After that, rather high correlations (between .55 and .75) were obtained, the highest for 70% of maximum. The retest correlations for RPE $\times$ HR were of the same magnitude, except at 100%, where it was .86. These retest correlations must be considered very high since they were calculated for each workload and not for selected loads from light to heavy. A correlation coefficient calculated on data from a large range of intensities can therefore be estimated to be above .90.

In a study by Borg, Karlsson, and Ekelund (1977) 20 male subjects were tested on a bicycle ergometer with two different tests, one in which HR guided the loads and one in which RPE guided the loads. All subjects performed the tests with a week of rest between them. A retest correlation was calculated on the workload that the subjects rated 17 on the two different tests. A correlation of .89 was obtained, which must be regarded high since not only was there a time delay between the two tests, but also two very different protocols were used.

In a study performed by Lamb (1995) a new test, the Children's Effort Rating Table (CERT), was compared with the RPE scale. Seventy school children were randomly assigned to one of two groups and tested on the bicycle ergometer with either RPE or CERT. They were retested after seven days. The study showed that both scales were very reliable, with a retest correlation for CERT of .91 and for RPE .90. Correlations were somewhat higher with HR for CERT, and Lamb concludes that CERT might be of great value for monitoring perceived exertion in children. Since this is the first and only study of CERT and only

a very rough description of the scale construction is given (the selection of verbal anchors and their positions on the scale is unclear), it is difficult to make any more positive statements about the value of CERT.

In a study by Eston and Williams (1988) retest reliability of the RPE scale was tested five to seven days apart. A pretest measured maximal oxygen uptake. The subjects then cycled at constant work rates based on their perception of intensities corresponding to RPE 9, 13, and 17. Between-trial correlations for $\dot{V}O_2$ were highest for visits 2 and 3 at RPE levels 9 and 13 (.83 and .94) and consistently high ($r = .92$ or greater) for the trials at RPE 17. The authors conclude that the RPE scale is a useful method for regulating high levels of exercise intensity in healthy men and women.

## Reliability Estimates From Validity Coefficients

A special approach to estimate reliability coefficients is to utilize obtained validity coefficients. This approach lends strong support that the reliability of measurements obtained with the RPE scale must be at least .90. This conclusion is drawn from the knowledge about the effect of attenuation and the size of the validity coefficients. The general equation for attenuation is

$$r_{TG} = r_{tg} / \sqrt{r_{tt} \cdot r_{gg}}$$

where $r_{TG}$ is the "true" (without errors in test and criterion) correlation, $r_{tg}$ is the obtained correlation, and $r_{tt}$ and $r_{gg}$ show the reliability of the test and the criterion, respectively. The coefficient $r_{TG}$ can hardly be higher than .90 because of the similarities and differences of the attributes RPE and HR and because both cannot perfectly measure the variable "exercise intensity." (For example, several other physiological and psychological variables referring to different aerobic and anaerobic factors, emotion, motivation, and personality, including rating behavior, should be measured and integrated.) With obtained validity correlations around .85 and HR reliabilities as high as .96, we obtain

$$.90 = .85 / \sqrt{r_{tt} \cdot .96}$$

and thus

$$r_{tt} = (.85 / .90)^2 \cdot 1 / .96 = .93$$

This reliability coefficient (.93) is probably not too high an estimate when the RPE scale is used in tests aimed at measuring exercise intensity. Validity coefficients higher than .85 have been obtained, especially when RPE values have been correlated with relative HR values, that is, when HR is corrected according to position in individual ranges.

Summarizing the studies on reliability, we can conclude that very high coefficients have been obtained, most above .90. An objection to retest coefficients is that subjects may remember what ratings they have given before and thus cause a spuriously high coefficient. However, the correlation is at the same time decreased because subjects are performing slightly differently or are in a slightly different condition during the second test. Remember that the reliability is not in a simple and constant way inherent in an instrument, but depends on the measurements obtained with an instrument. And the measurements depend greatly on exercise mode, context, and type of population tested. The very high correlations between RPE and HR show that the reliability must be very high in well-controlled ergometer situations; certainly about .92 or higher. This means that the error of method expressed as a percentage of the mean value is not more than 6%.

# Validity of the Scale

In the psychometric test tradition, validity is a very fundamental concept. Within psychophysics, however, validity has not been recognized as a major problem. The assessment of perceptual intensities and their validity depend greatly on the procedure used in obtaining the responses. Given a good definition of the attribute to be measured, a reliable method, and instruction that is precise, it is thought that high validity is ensured. The content of the questions to be asked (e.g., "How sour is this lemon?" or "How heavy is this stone?") and the construction of the method of assessment provide a natural, built-in validity. There is no direct, "outer" criterion to which the subjective responses can be correlated.

Content and construct validity are being used increasingly in psychometric studies, especially with tests of personality states or traits. In a suitable test situation, with good instruction, a well-motivated individual, and so on, a verbal report has to be considered true or the best estimate we can get. If the individual is doing his or her best

and there are no reasons to suspect his or her motives, the judgment must be taken for granted. If an individual claims that he or she has some pain or that a certain movement provokes aches of a special kind, there is no way to verify this objectively.

In the psychophysical tradition the internal consistency of judgments is therefore of primary interest. A fundamental theoretical assumption behind the ratio scaling methods is that equal stimulus ratios produce equal response ratios. Methods such as ratio setting (e.g., halving and doubling) and magnitude estimation are considered valid because they are designed to be ratio scaling methods. The fact that it is possible to describe sensation growth with one and the same kind of mathematical function (e.g., power function) for most perceptual modalities supports the generalizability of these methods. However, a drawback with ratio scaling methods that Stevens and collaborators never fully understood was their lack of validity in terms of direct determinations of intensity levels and interindividual comparisons (see S.S. Stevens 1971, 1975; Borg 1982a, 1992, 1994b; Sagal and Borg 1993).

The validity of the RPE scale was, to begin with, shown by its content and construction. By starting from common experiences, common sense, and judgments given by many healthy people and patients performing heavy physical tasks during leisure-time activities or during an exercise test, many different sensations and symptoms were collected. Among the different sensations were those originating from the muscles and joints involved in the performance, somatosensory sensations of pressure and strain, sensations of heat and sweating, and sensations from the chest region, especially breathlessness but also aches and pain for some people. Further sensations were those from the inner organs (e.g., from the stomach), feeling sick, or dizziness. The major sensation components or cues in healthy people were those coming from the working muscles and the chest (especially respiration).

In the first studies of perceived exertion using a bicycle ergometer, it was natural to instruct the subject to rate the exertion, effort, and fatigue that were perceived during the test and that were related to the exercise intensity. This kind of operational definition constituted the meaning and validity of the ratings. For different people, different cues might have dominated: for some leg exertion, for some breathlessness, and for some patients also pain.

# Content Validity

Chapter 1 gives the constitutional meaning of perceived exertion. Like concepts such as subjective force and heaviness, it is easy to understand and well anchored in common language. The construction of the RPE scale and the instruction for the scale captures the meaning of the words and the sensory perceptions that the words stand for. The scale makes it possible to measure the intensity of perceived exertion in a way that most people can agree on.

A measurement of perceived exertion refers to an individual's inner state and the intensity that this state has in the individual's frame of reference. Thus, it does not primarily depend on a position in a certain class of objects and events (e.g., the heaviness of a vase) but on the more "absolute" inner feeling.

The correspondence between observer ratings of perceived exertion and self-ratings are also good. The correspondence is similar to that between judgments of heaviness given by people lifting heavy objects and judgments by others observing them doing the work. The psychomotor movement pattern and the body language of the person performing the task tells the observer about the relative heaviness, which depends on the actual weight and the strength of the subject. Human perception is astonishingly good at revealing this heaviness directly, quickly, and spontaneously. This is in agreement with the Gibsonian tradition (Gibson 1979) as studied by Runesson and Frykholm (1981). As shown by Hueting during the congress of the International Association of Applied Psychology in Amsterdam in 1968, it is possible to estimate the degree of perceived exertion even from simple color slides of people using a bicycle ergometer.

In a study by Ljunggren (1986) observer ratings and self-ratings were collected for exercise on a bicycle ergometer and correlated with each other. Very high correlations were obtained for ratings given over a range of power levels, with $r_{xy} = .96$ for magnitude estimation, and $r_{xy} = .98$ for a scale similar to the CR10 scale.

# Construct Validity

Perceived exertion is a measurable variable when it is tied to a measuring instrument, such as the RPE scale or the CR10 scale. The construction of the RPE scale is very special since it results in ratings during an ergometer test with a stepwise increase of the workload; the ratings grow linearly with the load (see Borg 1977; Borg and Ottoson 1986). Theoretically, since the energy demand grows linearly with power, the subjective responses on the scale may do so also.

This general S-R relationship should also be found for different individuals. Differences between individuals, to a great extent, then possibly should be explained by differences in fundamental physical demands. According to the range model, the absolute values in the form of $\dot{V}O_2$ or absolute exercise intensity should correlate rather well with RPE, but not as well as individualized measurements, that is, measurements corrected for working capacity. The theoretical foundation of the construct of perceived exertion—and RPE as a measure mainly of exercise intensity—implies that high correlations can be obtained with simultaneously measured physiological criteria of exercise intensity (concurrent validity) and with predicted performance criteria. Perceived exertion, however, should also leave room for correlations with some psychological measurements reflecting emotional and motivational aspects of performance.

# Concurrent Validity

When studying perceived exertion during heavy exercise, measurements of physiological responses are often collected simultaneously. This offers good opportunities for obtaining correlations between perceptual and physiological responses. I don't think there is any other field in psychology in which measurements of a mental attribute can be correlated to so many relevant physiological variables. This does not mean, however, that there are any simple cause-effect relationships. Even if much of the variance in perceptual estimates can theoretically be "explained" by physiological cues, there are other important factors contributing to the variance; look on the cues from exercise physiology mainly as important correlates.

As previously pointed out, the concept of perceived exertion and the construction of the RPE scale mean that higher correlations should be obtained with physiological variables measuring relative exercise intensity than with those measuring absolute intensity (Borg 1977; Pandolf 1983). Since HR is a good measure of relative exercise intensity, many studies have used correlations between RPE and HR as evidence of concurrent validity.

The linearly increasing growth function between RPE, $\dot{V}O_2$, and HR is a *general* validation of the scale. High correlations between RPE and physiological variables across subjects show the scale's validity as a *differential* test (test of individual differences). Studies done in Umeå, Sweden, in 1966 to 1967 showed high correlations between RPE and HR similar to those previously obtained with the old 21-grade scale. In experiments carried out by Noble and Sherman in 1967, and by Bar-Or, Buskirk, and Skinner in 1968, these high correlations were further cross-validated.

In the first of three experiments performed from 1967 to 1968, results from an exercise test on the bicycle ergometer (according to Sjöstrand with stepwise increasing loads) showed a correlation between RPE and HR of .94. For a randomized-order test the correlation was .88, and for a treadmill test it was .85. The correlations between RPE and HR for a constant load were, however, rather low, for example, .46 for 100 W (Borg, Sherman, and Noble 1968).

The second study (Skinner et al. 1973) confirmed the linear relationship between RPE, workload, and HR, revealing a high correlation between these variables, $r_{xy} = .90$. In the third study (Bar-Or et al. 1972) 70 subjects between 41 and 60 years of age took part in an experiment both on the bicycle ergometer and the treadmill. RPE values were collected, together with some physiological measurements. The correlation coefficients between HR and RPE were .77 and .80, respectively.

In another study (Borg 1972) 28 subjects completed a test on a bicycle ergometer and provided RPE values, HR, and percentage estimates of perceived exertion (with a conceived maximal intensity as point of reference). At the lowest workloads the correlations were low or insignificant. At 100 W the correlation was .31 for percentage ratings and HR, and .65 for RPE and HR. At 150 W the corresponding correlations were .56 and .68. For the whole work test (with subjects randomly selected from different loads) the correlation was .80 for percentage ratings and somewhat higher, .86, for RPE and HR.

The RPE scale has been translated to many different languages. Using a translation to Hebrew, a large study was performed at the Wingate Institute in Israel (Bar-Or 1977). Thirteen groups of subjects from 7 to 68 years of age (a total of 1,316 subjects) were tested on a bicycle ergometer in nine different projects. The highest correlations between HR and RPE (.70 to .90) were

obtained for the teenagers. The correlations dropped as subjects' age increased and were lowest for the oldest group of physically active men 50 to 68 years old ($r_{xy} = .60$). (The decrease in correlation values with age may be due to smaller ranges in HR and subjects' more homogeneous working capacity.)

A German study by Ulmer, Janz, and Löllgen (1977) obtained a correlation of .89 between RPE and HR for ergometer work, thus showing very high concurrent validity for the German version of the scale. In an ergometer study using the RPE scale translated into Japanese, Miyashita, Onodera, and Tabata (1986) examined a group of Japanese men and found a correlation of .84 between RPE and percentage of maximal HR and a correlation of .76 between RPE and percentage of $\dot{V}O_2$max. They also studied boys 7 to 18 years old and found low correlations (.55 to .74) for the youngest boys (7 to 9 years old), while most values obtained for the older age groups were higher than .90. These very high validity correlations between RPE and HR have been further cross-validated in several later investigations (see Borg 1977; Pandolf 1983; Borg and Ottoson 1986).

RPE values have also been correlated with other physiological measurements, such as $\dot{V}O_2$, ventilation measurements, blood lactates, and so on. Generally, these correlations have been somewhat lower than those for HR. Since RPE is an individualized measure of exercise intensity, it is natural that it should correlate better with measures of relative strain than with measures of physical stress, which assess absolute aerobic demands. Thus, the correlations between RPE and $\dot{V}O_2$ are often 10% to 20% lower than those between RPE and HR (Ulmer, Janz, and Löllgen 1977; Pandolf 1983).

The fact that RPE is an individualized measure of relative strain rather than absolute stress makes it of great interest in correlating RPE with relative HR values according to Karvonen or Borg's range model (Borg 1961a; Karvonen, Kentala, and Musta 1957). In a study by Pavlina and Saric (1975), such a correlation was done by testing subjects on the bicycle ergometer at submaximal exertion and also at maximal exertion to obtain actual measurements of maximal HR in an age-heterogeneous group of male subjects. The correlation between RPE and absolute HR was .90, while that between RPE and relative HR (HR reserve) was significantly higher, .94.

All of the studies reported in this section used healthy people as subjects. When people with diseases are included in the test group, the correlations between HR and RPE drop rather markedly. This was first shown by Borg and Linderholm (1970) with the old 21-grade scale. With the addition of subjects with health problems, the correlations dropped from about .85 to .50 or .70. This is quite natural since in patients with different diseases, other cues of both physiological and of psychological origin, such as pain and anxiety, may influence RPE and also HR, to some extent in different ways.

## Predictive Validity

The high validity coefficients reported in the preceding section on concurrent validity indicate that predictive validity should also be high. Sometimes concurrent validity is considered to be one part of predictive validity; that is, "predictions" are made about simultaneously obtained measurements. However, most often we want to know how well RPE can be used to predict something later in time. One of the most important things to predict is performance, especially maximal performance.

Several studies have shown that RPE may be used with great confidence for predicting performance. Using the old 21-grade scale Borg (1962a) predicted maximal cycling strength thresholds on the bicycle ergometer using previously obtained ratings from only one power level. For the ratings to be valid for such short-term work, a strong negative correlation should be obtained between the ratings and the maximal strength thresholds. This was the case in a group of 20 subjects (14 men and 6 women) 20 to 25 years old, who worked for half a minute at one power level, 330 W. The rank correlation obtained was very high, $r_s = -.83$. For work of longer duration on the bicycle ergometer, the predictive power for maximal performances was also found to be about as good as for HR (Borg 1962a).

These results, which show that measures of perceived exertion can be used to predict short-term performances (less than 1 min), to my knowledge have been cross-validated in only one study (Borg 1982a). In that study it was important to get a submaximal estimate of a maximal performance for half a minute in order to select the right intensity level for testing anaerobic capacity in a new cycling strength test (see chapter 8).

In collaboration with the Swedish army, 90 conscripts (men 18 to 19 years old) performed an aerobic test on the bicycle ergometer at a constant load of 230 W during a maximal time of 12 min. After 12 min the power was increased by 33 W for 6 min for those who could go on, then by another 33 W for 6 min, and so on, until everyone had finished. Thus, the time it took to finish the test gave an estimate of physical working capacity. The subjects rated the perceived exertion after the first minute and then every second minute. Correlations were calculated between submaximal ratings and time to finish the test. High correlations were obtained; after 1 min the correlation was −.56, and after 3 min it was −.72. Only half of the young men were able to pedal more than 7 min, but at that time the correlation was still −.66 in spite of the restricted range. The material was also analyzed in a different way by determining the time it took for the men to give a certain rating and correlating that with the time it took to finish. The correlation between time to finish and exercise time to elicit a rating of 13 was .60, for a rating of 15 it was .70, and for 17 it was .79. These correlations thus showed that it is quite possible to predict maximal exercise time from submaximal ratings (Borg 1966).

The fact that RPE can be used to predict maximal performances involving high aerobic demands has been shown in quite a few studies (e.g., see Borg and Ottoson 1986). RPE is often used like HR; that is, an estimate of working capacity is calculated from submaximal responses during a test with stepwise increments in intensity. The obtained $W_{HR}$ and the $W_{RPE}$ are highly correlated to actual measurements of working capacity, with coefficients of about .50 to .70 (see chapter 8).

## Further Comments About Validity

Most well-controlled experiments obtain high validity coefficients. Studies reporting low validity have commonly used a small group of subjects or a special selection of subjects with little exercise experience or low motivation to participate or to attend correctly to the cues for perceived exertion. Sometimes studies use a homogeneous group of subjects with regard to working capacity. In these cases, a rather low correlation between RPE and HR is obtained, especially if only a restricted range of exercise intensities has been used, resulting in little variation in both variables. Also, low correlations can be obtained when the group of subjects is heterogeneous with regard to physiological responses, for example, because of great age differences or different dysfunctions. Insufficient instruction may also cause low validity and reliability of the ratings because the subjects do not really know what to rate.

For exercise at low intensities there is quite a bit of "noise in the system" when it comes to both physiological responses and sensory perceptions. HR and RPE at rest or at very low intensities is rather variable across subjects, and emotional factors also may have great influence. Factors in the environment, such as music, heat, and social context, may distract subjects or cause them to attend to special cues, resulting in their selection of a rating that is too high or too low.

At very high exercise intensities close to maximum, the correlation between RPE and HR cannot be expected to be high. There are rather large differences among subjects in maximal HR and also in maximal RPE, resulting in a low correlation between these variables. Some subjects may also experience aches and pain, breathing diffi-

culties, or anxiety about a possible overload at high intensities. The latter factor is most important when testing patients who are afraid to exercise and therefore unconsciously or intentionally give a rating that is too high. It may be necessary to retest this group of patients and give them additional instructions about the importance of the test and about being as unbiased and realistic as possible. It may also be a good idea to give them some control over the exercise intensity. This may be done by letting them set a preferred resistance and then increasing it in small steps that they can learn to tolerate.

Construction of psychophysical scales is an ongoing scientific process. The Borg RPE scale is an example of a successful scale construction for a specific purpose. Other scales are needed in certain cases, however, as a complement to the Borg RPE scale for perceived exertion and for scaling other attributes, such as aches and pain. I present the Borg CR10 scale in the next chapter. It is a special scale with different psychometric properties than the RPE scale.

---

## Is Gardening Effortful?

From personal experience, I know that some subjects, even those whom one might expect to give valid ratings, find it difficult to understand the task. I remember once asking my neighbor, an intelligent and strong man who was a colonel in the army, how hard he perceived gardening to be when he worked at it rather hard. He answered that he didn't exert himself at all. I was astonished and tried to get him to respond differently, but he insisted that this kind of work "is not exertion." I obtained a similar response from a friend of my wife when I asked her how sour she thought a lemon was. She answered, "I don't think a lemon is sour."

It seems as if some people do not want to categorize a sensory perception as strong unless it is very strong, or they allow the perceived intensity to be influenced by their preferences. A few people may think of exertion as a kind of "overexertion." For these people light exertion is no exertion at all. Light pain, on the other hand, is not as easy to miss or to evaluate positively as light exertion. I myself do not like standing still during a conversation, but prefer walking while talking. I have used this method for individual oral examinations of doctoral students. In this situation you can forget that you are walking and not perceive any exertion at all, at least no physical effort.

# Chapter 6

# The Borg CR10 Scale

Hundreds of studies have shown the RPE scale to function very well. The linearity between ratings, workload, and HR and the high correlation across subjects with HR and some other physiological variables in healthy people make it easy to use. In some situations, however, it is of interest to use a ratio scaling method, such as magnitude estimation (see chapter 4). This is the case particularly when it is important to be able to describe a psychophysical S-R function and its specific form over a wide range of intensities with a mathematical function that as accurately as possible reflects the genuine growth of the sensory perception. An example of this occurs when comparing S-R functions for different modalities and for perceptual and physiological reactions. In these cases it is necessary to try to control and measure not only the independent variables, but also the dependent variables (physical, physiological, and perceptual variables) with scales having the same (or as similar as possible) metric properties, preferably ratio scales.

However, when using a ratio scaling method the lack of an intersubjective unit for direct determinations of intensity levels causes disadvantages. Thus arose the idea to construct a *category-ratio scale*, with the advantages of a simple rating method for direct level estimates and the advantages of a ratio scaling method for determinations of ratio relationships between perceptual responses. With such a scale a researcher could determine both relative growth functions and absolute levels.

The Borg CR10 scale was constructed to meet these demands, but the principles behind the construction of the CR10 scale are somewhat different from those behind the construction of the RPE scale. The most fundamental difference is the demand of a nonlinear and positively accelerating growth function for the CR10 responses when scaling perceived exertion and possibly also pain. Some common properties between the scales are also needed, especially when it comes to their differential use at moderate to high intensities.

The reliability and validity of the measurements obtained with a scale depend greatly on the attribute to be scaled. Since the perception of effort and exertion is such an easily scalable attribute, individual differences can reliably be measured with both scales. Chapter 5's report on the RPE scale and comparisons with the old 21-grade and other scales show that high reliability coefficients may be obtained with several scales. This means that reliability is not a big problem for the CR10 scale either, since for differential use it has properties in common with the RPE scale, except for the most extreme intensities. A more pressing question is the validity of the growth functions.

## Construction of the Scale

Whereas the RPE scale was constructed to follow the physiologically linear increase of aerobic energy demands for increasing exercise intensity, no such reasons are evident when it comes to scaling pain. Instead there is some evidence that in several situations (depending on how the distal or proximal stimulus is identified) pain should increase according to a positively accelerating function (Price 1988). Pain is a very special attribute since (as discussed in chapter 2) most sensory perceptions merge into pain at the highest intensities; that is, the quality of sensation changes from, for example, loudness, sourness, heat, or cold to pain, and together with this change in quality comes a change in intensity, pain being much stronger than anything else. A person may experience a pain stronger than he or she has ever experienced before. People must therefore be able to respond with a number higher than expected according to previous experiences. It is thus important not to have a fixed endpoint, but to let the subject be free to choose a higher number than that anchored in an ordinary rating scale or the Visual Analog Scale (VAS).

There were several principles and considerations behind constructing the CR10 scale. The first and perhaps most fundamental principle was the range model previously described. The information obtained from studies in quantitative semantics showed that adjectives and adverbs may function as multiplicative constants and give good meanings for anchoring numbers (according to an inner frame of reference). Second, the knowledge gained from several psychophysiological studies on both perceived exertion and taste perception were important in constructing the CR10 scale (see Borg 1982a). Perceptual growth functions, together with psychophysiological growth functions, had been established with the use of both ratio scaling methods and rating scales with verbal anchors. Comparisons could therefore be made between these different functions, and special scale transformations could be performed. According to S.S. Stevens and Galanter (1957) a symmetrical cat-

egory rating scale is related to a ratio scale according to a special nonlinear function. In our studies on perceived exertion the same relationship was found, and it was therefore possible to change the position of the verbal anchors on the rating scale to a truer position on a ratio scale. The main idea behind the transformation is seen in figure 6.1.

I made a first attempt at constructing a category-ratio scale (that is, a combination of a category scale for direct level determinations and a ratio scale for determinations of scale tests and growth functions) in the early 1970s. Proceeding from most of the previously described considerations, I constructed a scale from 0 (absolutely no feeling at all of exertion) to 20 (maximal exertion). "Very light" was placed at 2, "somewhat hard" at 6, "hard" at 10, "very hard" at 14, and "very, very hard" at 18. The scale was tested in short-term ergometer work, and an exponent of 1.57 was obtained (similar to those previously obtained with ratio scaling methods; Borg 1973a). The scale was also presented during the first major international symposium on perceived exertion, "Physical Work and Effort," held at the Wenner-Gren Center, Stockholm, in 1975 (see Borg 1977).

The CR10 scale was constructed to simplify scaling for practical use and to improve scaling of the most extreme intensities—the "most intense pain sensation imaginable." It consisted of a limited number range from 0 to 0.5 to 1 to 10, with numbers placed at positions so that a linear relation could be obtained roughly with

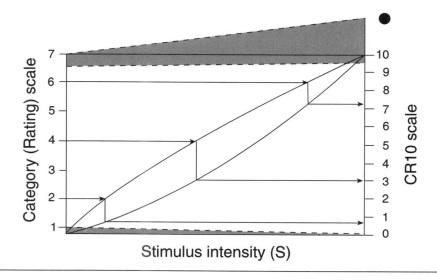

**Figure 6.1**  A schematic of the first steps in converting a category rating scale to a category-ratio (CR) scale.

> ## A Marriage Between a Cat and a Rat
>
> The fact that the CR10 scale is unique is not fully recognized by most people who use the scale. They perceive the relationship between numbers and verbal descriptors as a curious one and don't recognize the good harmony that exists between the increase indicated by the numbers and that denoted by the descriptors. Obtaining harmony between a category (C) scale and a ratio (R) scale is, however, as difficult as getting a cat and a rat to collaborate. Stevens condemned category scaling and felt that there was little to justify its use. He hoped that category scaling would disappear but "hoped in vain" (S.S. Stevens 1971). Others—such as Parducci, who called it "the pipeline to the psyche"—have defended category scaling. Experimental studies in animal conditioning have shown that it is possible to get a cat to collaborate with a rat. And our experiments in psychophysical scaling have clearly demonstrated the advantages of taking the best properties of a category scale and combining them with the best properties of a ratio scale to make a "cat-rat" scale such as the CR10.

data from magnitude estimation. To avoid bottom and ceiling effects and to make the scale more finely graded, the new scale was constructed (by iterative methods and extrapolations of the monotonous function), and its instruction encouraged ratings with decimals below 0.5, between the anchors, and also above 10, such as 11 or 12 or even higher. The rating 10 was anchored as "extremely strong" perceived exertion, corresponding to the most intense perception of effort and exertion a person has ever experienced before (see figure 6.2). A slight modification is now made to encourage responses of 1.5, 2.5, and above 10 up to "maximal" (see chapter 7, figure 7.4).

| 0 | Nothing at all | |
|------|-------------------|------------------|
| 0.5 | Extremely weak | (just noticeable) |
| 1 | Very weak | |
| 2 | Weak | (light) |
| 3 | Moderate | |
| 4 | | |
| 5 | Strong | (heavy) |
| 6 | | |
| 7 | Very strong | |
| 8 | | |
| 9 | | |
| 10 | Extremely strong | (almost max) |
| ● | Maximal | |

Borg CR10 scale
© Gunnar Borg, 1981, 1982

**Figure 6.2** The old Borg CR10 scale, a category (C) scale with ratio (R) properties for most perceptual continua.

My daughter and I (Borg and Borg 1994) have constructed other CR scales (e.g., CR100, the CentiMax [CM] Scale) according to the same CR principles as used for the CR10 scale but changed them to be even more finely graded. They have been tested on some perceptual continua, such as perceived exertion, blackness, taste, and loudness (Marks, Borg, and Ljunggren 1983; Borg, Ljunggren, and Marks 1985; Borg and Borg 1994), and found to function well. There is no major difference between different CR scales, but since the CR10 scale is very reliable and easy to use—with good instruction and suitable training material—it has become more popular than other CR scales.

## Reliability of the Scale

In most studies on perceived exertion similar reliability coefficients have been obtained with both the CR10 and the RPE scales. Both scales have been used in connection with teaching and training at our laboratory and correlate highly with each other and with HR. In a study by Ljunggren and Johansson (1988) reliability coefficients (using CR10) were determined for ratings of perceived exertion ($R_e$) and for ratings of pain ($R_p$) during a bicycle ergometer test and compared to those for heart rate (HR) and blood lactate (BL). The split-half correlations (Spearman-Brown) were $R_e = .96$, $R_p = .96$, HR $= .97$, and BL $= .98$. The correlation between power levels corresponding to the ratings $R_{e5}$, $R_{e7}$ and $R_{p5}$, $R_{p7}$ were also very high: $W_{Re5} \times W_{Re7} = .87$ and $W_{Rp5} \times W_{Rp7} = .95$. A repeated-measures design gave correlations

---

## The First CR Scale

In 1975 I organized an international symposium on work and effort at the Wenner-Gren Center in Stockholm. One of the leading psychophysicists, Dr. William Cane from Yale, proposed the idea of combining the advantages of ratio scaling techniques with those of simple category rating methods by placing verbal anchors at the appropriate positions. I was then happy to respond that I had already done so, having experimented with and constructed the first category-ratio scale for perceived exertion (Borg 1973a; see also Borg 1977).

---

around .92. These reliability coefficients are all very satisfactory.

In a study of the reliability of self-ratings for hand-arm vibrations, Wos and co-workers (1988) collected ratings of the perceived vibration for different frequencies and intensity levels. They used the CR10 scale, calculated several different reliability coefficients, and found that most were around .90. They summarized their results by saying that the coefficients are high: "0.986 for experienced subjects and .841 for inexperienced subjects."

Harms-Ringdahl and collaborators at the Karolinska Hospital in Stockholm have been using different scales to assess pain and other symptoms both clinically on various groups of patients with musculoskeletal disorders and experimentally on healthy subjects. In one study (Harms-Ringdahl et al. 1986) the reliability of the CR10 scale was determined by comparing it with the Visual Analog Scale (VAS) that previously had been found reliable for assessments of subjective strain and pain. Load-elicited pain was provoked in healthy subjects by stressing passive joint structures in the arm (elbow). The subjects rated the pain on one of the scales at a time in different sessions on different days with the scales in randomized order. Individual correlations were calculated and found to be rather high, with a variation over subjects from .78 to .99 (mean .90). These correlations must be regarded as high since the determinations involved both a parallel-testing and a retest design.

In a study by Neely (1995) CR scaling was compared with other scaling methods and was found to work equally well or better than the others. In a separate study (Neely et al. 1992) responses obtained with the CR10 scale were compared with those obtained with VAS. For ratings of perceived exertion collected with the two scales, correlations from .79 to .97 were obtained for different workloads. Retest correlations were .98 and .85. Since these correlations refer only to separate workloads, they are very high and indicate that if responses had been collected from a wide range of workloads, much higher correlations may have been obtained. If we express the reliability in the form of a percentage error of the mean value for a standard deviation of 1.5 and a mean rating level of 7, we obtain a measurement error of about 6%.

The correlations between HR and CR10 are slightly lower than those between HR and RPE. This may be due to two factors: the nonlinearity to HR and the slightly smaller numerical range for the most common intensities, from "very weak" ("very light") to "very strong" ("very hard"). The CR10 scale ranges from 1 to 7 in this span, and the RPE scale from 9 to 17 (seven scale steps for the CR10 scale and nine for the RPE scale).

# Validity of the Scale

The content validity of the CR10 scale is secured by the definitions, the instructions, and the testing contexts with relation to perceived exertion and the RPE scale and to pain and the VAS.

The construct validity of special interest for this scale concerns the perceptual growth function and the similarities and differences to other scaling methods. The CR10 scale is constructed to give a general increase in sensory perceptions of the same kind as those obtained with ratio scaling methods (magnitude estimation). The validity of the scale in this general sense has been shown in several studies. Power functions describe the relative growth functions with exponents just slightly lower than those obtained in studies on perceived exertion, taste, blackness, and loudness, using magnitude estimation (Borg and Borg 1994).

In a study on the bicycle ergometer the CR10 scale was used to measure both leg effort, chest effort, and leg pain as well as the physiological correlates (HR, blood lactate, and muscle lactate; Noble et al. 1983). All the subjective variables showed positively accelerated functions with similar exponents (1.63 to 1.67) but the leg pain function was lower than the others (showing a general, lower intensity manifested in a lower measurement constant). The perceptual variables followed functions between those for the increase of HR and lactate. While HR increases rather linearly with power, both lactate functions can be described by monotonously increasing power functions with exponents 2.2 (blood lactate) and 2.7 (muscle lactate). A similar study by Borg, Ljunggren, and Ceci (1985) found the same exponent for effort (1.63) but about 2 for pain (1.98). The pain curve more closely followed the function for blood lactate (2.98, also a monotonously increasing power function).

Borg et al. (1987) studied the relationships between RPE, HR, blood lactate, and category-ratio values for three different exercise modes; these relationships are shown in table 6.1. It is very interesting to see in table 6.1 how well the interrelationships among the dependent variables agree. There is an *invariance of relations,* so that when one mode of exercise is changed all exponents change proportionally. The variation in CR values can be predicted rather simply from a combination of HR and blood lactate.

When the CR10 scale is used to measure perceived exertion, correlation coefficients showing validity of the measurements are of a similar magnitude as those for the RPE scale. The concurrent validity based on correlations between simultaneously collected ratings and HR is high in several studies. In a study by Ljunggren (1985) the correlation between cyclists' own ratings of exertion and their HR was .91. When observers rated the cyclists' exertion, the corresponding correlation was .79, and when the observers saw the cyclists only on video tape without any sound, it was still rather high (.68).

**Table 6.1.** General Functions (Exponents) of Intensity Indicators for Cycling, Running, and Walking

| Indicator | Cycling | Running | Walking |
|---|---|---|---|
| Heart rate | 1.0 | 1.0 | 2.0 |
| Blood lactate | 2.5 | 2.5 | ≥3.0 |
| Ratio scaling | 1.6 | 1.6 | 3.0 |
| RPE | 1.0 | 1.0 | 2.0 |

A study by Marks, Borg, and Ljunggren (1983) collected both magnitude estimations (ME) and CR responses (according to a scale only slightly different from the CR10) during ergometer exercise. Correlations between ratings and HR for a low power level (65 W) were .10 for ME and .50 for CR. At a rather high level (163 W) they were .24 for ME and .66 for CR. These correlations between CR and HR must be considered very high since they were calculated on responses from constant loads. All ME coefficients were statistically insignificant.

A study published in a Swedish report series by Åhsberg and Gamberale (1996) presented a new instrument for evaluating perceptions of fatigue during physical work. For ergometer work, ratings with the new instrument correlated .94 with HR. Ratings with CR10 were slightly higher, as high as .96. The corresponding correlations with systolic blood pressure were .79 and .78, respectively.

Predictive validity based on correlations between CR10 ratings and performances is also rather high. The validity of $W_R$ measurements (e.g., $W_{R7}$ calculated from the plot of CR ratings to workloads [W] using 7 on the scale as level of reference) in the form of correlations between $W_R$ and $W_{max}$ (maximal working capacity) was clearly significant, the highest being the one between $W_{R7}$ and $W_{max}$ ($r_{xy}$ = .56; Ljunggren and Johansson 1988).

The CR10 scale is now used in an increasing number of studies of pain, both laboratory studies on experimental pain in healthy subjects and clinical studies on patients. Researchers using the CR10 scale and comparing the results with other methods report good validity. The most convincing evidence of the CR10 scale's validity is the very high correlations between CR10 and VAS (see Neely 1995) because VAS is already generally accepted by the International Association for the Study of Pain as a valid scale for pain assessments. The advantage of CR10 over VAS is the CR10 scale's ability to discriminate among the most extreme and maximal intensities and to facilitate communication. The validity of CR10 ratings is also shown by their discriminative power in clinical diagnostics and in ergonomic evaluations of different work tasks as reported in part III concerning specific applications of the Borg RPE and Borg CR10 scales.

# Chapter 7

# Administration of the Borg Scales

In terms of theories and standards, much of the knowledge about administration of ordinary psychometric tests can be applied in psychophysical scaling. Reports obtained from scaling can be looked on as samples reflecting people's specific sensations and experiences in certain situations. To permit valid generalizations the test situation and the response methodology must be well standardized.

## General Principles

Information that covers most of the important aspects of scale administration should include the four W's and the two H's: why?, what?, where?, when?, and how to rate?, and how to evaluate? The test subject must know why we are doing this test, where and when it is going to take place, what we will be doing, what we want him or her to rate, and, not least, how it is going to be done.

In most situations in which scaling is applied, good preparation and general instructions are important first steps, not only for the application of my scales, but also for most kinds of physiological and psychological tests. One of the most important requirements is good preparation before the test, including preparation of the test leader, the situation, and the subject. The test leader must have a good grasp of test methods and facts and must understand the purpose of the test, the procedure, the demands of standardization, and so on. The test leader must establish a good rapport with the person to be tested, acquaint him or her with the situation, and give all the relevant and necessary information.

Much can be said about test administration. However, there are so many different kinds of tests and training situations—laboratory or field testing contexts; leisure-time activities or specific work tasks of ergonomic, sport, or clinical interest; samples of healthy individuals or patients with diseases of different severity; purposes for scaling; and so on—that no single approach to administration can take all these different variables into account. Still, there are some general rules and specific instructions that should always be followed.

## Why: The Purpose of the Test

The subject often will find it natural that the test leader ask questions about perceived exertion, pain, or other subjective somatic symptoms during a test. However, it is still important to give a short explanation of why questions about subjective feelings during the tests are essential. Most often this explanation can be very simple and can include some general statements such as these: During the test we want you to rate your perception of exertion (or pain, etc.) because your own perception is an important complement to the physiological measurements we are going to take (these, of course, must be explained separately).

## What to Rate

What to rate is often simple to understand, depending on the purpose and the situation in question. However, it is still necessary to give good instructions with further explanations for rating both perceived exertion and pain. (Specific instructions appear later in this chapter.)

It is of special importance that the person tested understand that we want to scale his or her own perception as a subjective phenomenon. The test subject should attend to his or her inner subjective feelings and not think about the physical tasks or the physiological cues or responses. It is important that the subject try to be spontaneous and "naïve" and take an introspective, rather than a stimulus-oriented, approach. It is also important not to listen to or try to figure out what other people might think and say in a similar situation; instead the test subject should trust his or her own feelings.

## Where and When: The Test Situation

In field situations and clinical settings many factors may interfere with the desired conditions. The physical environment may be difficult to control and social factors may also be disturbing. Unfamiliar apparatus and scary instruments, music or noise, temperature, and the presence of other people and other activities may influence the performance and the rating. Such factors must be controlled to the greatest possible extent. However, if control is not possible, these factors must be accounted for when interpreting the results. In many laboratory situations it is rather easy to maintain rigid control over all influencing factors. Careful preparation of the situation before the test is necessary for a good result. Distracting stimuli, including other people coming into the test room, must be avoided. Even under well-controlled conditions, undesired things may happen, and all unusual testing conditions must be observed and reported.

The decision of when to test a person is often determined by physiological and medical factors and by the purpose of the test. When using RPE in tests of working capacity, the person should be well rested and alert and have followed his or her usual daily routine. The person should not be tested soon after intake of food or any drugs (unless absolutely necessary). Determinations of pain, however, must often be performed according to the special clinical, diagnostic, or therapeutic situation. Psychological factors also affect the ratings of perceived exertion and pain, and it is important to choose a time when the person is not too anxious, but calm and relaxed and—if possible—has a feeling of control over his or her situation.

The purpose of the test may make it necessary to choose a specific time and place. If the aim is to study the effect of special circumstances, such as diurnal rhythm, alcohol, or medication, the administration has to be fitted to these circumstances.

## How to Rate and How to Evaluate

To standardize the test procedure, a special psychophysical scale should be used. Explain this to the individual, and refer to the separate instructions later in this chapter.

An adequate scale instruction that is simple, clear, and easy to understand must be given to the individual. The instruction should not be too short or too long. It should include a short explanation of what to rate, how the scale functions, and what the verbal anchors mean. It should also include a short description of what is expected of the test subject and how important it is that he or she tries to be a good rater. No anchors other than those in the instruction and the verbal descriptors on the scale should be presented!

Again, the administration of a test and scaling of subjective somatic symptoms should follow a standardized procedure. However, depending on the person being tested, it may be necessary to adapt the instruction and provide further explanations and clarifications. It is very important that the test leader and the test subject have a good rapport and can collaborate. The administration should be controlled not only objectively, but also so that all subjects' understanding of and reaction to the situation is similar. Of course, to achieve good similarity an objectively standardized situation is the most important factor. However, because of different personality factors and unexpected situational factors, the test leader also must be competent enough to be flexible and allow some modifications.

Laboratory studies with students as subjects should seldom present any problems. However, testing patients with severe diseases may be more difficult. Some patients may have difficulties understanding the instructions, and it may be necessary to ask them about their experiences from certain daily activities, for example, how it feels to walk a short distance at their own preferred pace or to walk up stairs at home, what symptoms they have, what their memories of traumatic situations are, and so on. It is, of course, important to know beforehand what their main disabilities are in order to ask the right questions. It may also be necessary after a short period of testing to interrupt the test, clarify the instructions, then start again.

If necessary, it is always possible to check the rating behavior of the person by asking further questions that involve not only tasks associated with perceived exertion and pain, but many different kinds of experiences, for example, how sour he or she perceives a lemon to be, how white a piece of sugar is, how hot a cup of newly brewed coffee is, and so on. Special test material for evaluating rating behavior, sometimes used in connection with the CR10 scale, is now under further development.

Emotional factors, such as test anxiety, may influence the responses. Healthy subjects with compulsory neurotic traits commonly perceive a new and unfamiliar test situation as threatening. They display anxiety reactions with some increases in physiological responses (e.g., heart rate and blood pressure). A heart patient or a patient with lung disease or exercise-induced asthma may be anxious about exercising or undergoing other treatment and may respond with ratings that are too high. All these emotional responses have to be handled carefully; and in special cases, if the test leader is not a trained psychologist, he or she may have to collaborate with a clinical specialist. The test leader also can let subjects rate their actual mood state, such as degree of anxiety, emotional stress, depression, or discomfort using the CR10 scale.

Closely connected with emotional factors are motivational ones. Athletes commonly give underestimations of perceived exertion. Many athletes want to show that they are very fit and do not want to admit that they are exerting themselves as much as they actually are. The opposite may be the case for people who have low motivation to take part in the test. They do not see why they should exert themselves or they may want to pretend that they are less fit than they actually are. When subjects rate pain, similar motivational factors may influence the ratings. Cultural factors, suffering, and the meaning of pain in each person's psychosocial context must also be taken into consideration.

In these and other cases in which the subject does not collaborate well because of misunderstanding, anxiety, or low motivation, it may be necessary to spend time on an extended interview and explain how important it is to perform according to the instructions. The test leader can try to get the subject more involved in the testing (e.g., by letting the patient himself or herself increase the stimulus intensity) so that he or she can feel in control of the situation.

## Response Protocol

It is important to have a good protocol for recording the answers and other responses during the test. Special observations, both behavioral and physiological, may be important for the later evaluation—or for immediate emergency actions. If the responses are recorded directly on a computer, rather than in writing, it is important to check that no input errors are made!

# The Borg RPE Scale

The general principles presented so far should be followed together with the specific instructions for the RPE scale. It is especially important to plan what the subject is going to rate well before the test.

## What to Rate

The test instructions include an explanation of what perceived exertion is. Sometimes we want only an overall rating of perceived exertion as a kind of integration or gestalt of all the different exercise symptoms from the peripheral working muscles and joints and of sensations from the chest region. Sometimes we want to discriminate between different kinds of perceptions. For normal, healthy people we may want to obtain ratings of breathlessness, and of local exertion and fatigue from the working muscles involved. For patients, the sensations from the chest region can be separated into heart pain, normal breathlessness (panting), or abnormal breathing difficulties (dyspnea). For ergonomic work tasks the test subject may be instructed to attend specifically to the strain and difficulty of certain work operations.

The test subject must understand that it is not the physical difficulty (e.g., what the weight is or how warm it is) that counts, but the inner feeling of exertion, strain, and fatigue. A firefighter may experience a moderate degree of exertion but a strong degree of heat. He or she should then focus on the physical effort and fatigue and not on the degree of warmness (which he or she may do separately). Nor should the subject attend to the actual heart rate or respiratory rate. Trying to attend to physiological responses is as detrimental to the scaling as trying to figure out what the physical load is; instead, the test person should concentrate on the subjective feeling. Some subjects have difficulties with this and want to concentrate on the stimulus and the "real stress." They then commit a "stimulus error" by attending to the distal stimulus, such as the workload, or the proximal stimulus, represented by respiratory rate.

The following instructions should be given in an ordinary exercise test. For other kinds of work tasks and situations some minor variations may be necessary, but once again, the subject must not be instructed to attend to any distal or proximal stimuli.

## The RPE Scale

The original RPE scale (Borg 1970b) was slightly modified in the middle of the 1980s (Borg 1985). The revised scale is shown in figure 7.1.

---

### Scale Instructions

While exercising we want you to rate your perception of exertion, i.e., how heavy and strenuous the exercise feels to you. The perception of exertion depends mainly on the strain and fatigue in your muscles and on your feeling of breathlessness or aches in the chest.

Look at this rating scale; we want you to use this scale from 6 to 20, where 6 means "no exertion at all" and 20 means "maximal exertion."

| | |
|---|---|
| 6 | No exertion at all |
| 7 | |
| 8 | Extremely light |
| 9 | Very light |
| 10 | |
| 11 | Light |
| 12 | |
| 13 | Somewhat hard |
| 14 | |
| 15 | Hard (heavy) |
| 16 | |
| 17 | Very hard |
| 18 | |
| 19 | Extremely hard |
| 20 | Maximal exertion |

Borg RPE/ scale
© Gunnar Borg, 1970, 1985, 1994, 1998

---

**Figure 7.1**  The Borg RPE scale for perceived exertion.

9     corresponds to "very light" exercise. For a normal, healthy person it is like walking slowly at his or her own pace for some minutes.

13    on the scale is "somewhat hard" exercise, but it still feels OK to continue.

17    "very hard" is very strenuous. A healthy person can still go on, but he or she really has to push him- or herself. It feels very heavy, and the person is very tired.

19    on the scale is an extremely strenuous exercise level. For most people this is the most strenuous exercise they have ever experienced.

Try to appraise your feeling of exertion as honestly as possible, without thinking about what the actual physical load is. Don't underestimate it, but don't overestimate it either. It's your own feeling of effort and exertion that's important, not how it compares to other people's. What other people think is not important either. Look at the scale and the expressions and then give a number.

Any questions?

After the instruction is given, it is important that the test leader encourage the person to ask questions.

Psychophysical scaling sometimes uses special material to instruct and train the subject and maybe even to correct given responses. This is generally not necessary when using the RPE scale. The scale is constructed to be easy to use, and there is no need for any special instructional material. RPE has become a general term for ratings of perceived exertion, not only those obtained with this scale. It is therefore necessary in all studies to record explicitly what scale has been used, for example, "RPE was determined with the Borg RPE scale (Borg 1970b or Borg 1985), and the instruction given by Borg (Borg 1985)."

## How to Evaluate

RPE is a good complement to HR. As with HR, an RPE response is difficult to evaluate in a simple objective way in all situations. There are so many different kinds of tests, daily work situations, populations of healthy subjects and patients, contexts, and so on that no simple tables can summarize the meaning of an RPE response. Refer to part III, in which results from many different applications are given. For more information, see other books and research articles listed in the references at the end of this book.

The verbal descriptors (anchors) of the scale are chosen from ordinary, everyday language, with words that everyone should understand well. This means that for most people and most situations the anchors have a natural meaning that is built into the scale. The most common application of the RPE scale is to make comparisons not between but within individuals. These kinds of intraindividual comparisons have a direct and simple meaning for most individuals, since the people are their own controls. Thus, if someone has a tendency to give slightly high or low ratings, it has little effect on intraindividual comparisons in testing, training, and rehabilitation. It is important, however, that each individual understand the meaning of his or her response. In a rehabilitation program, for example, this understanding can be ensured simply by testing a patient and training him or her to rate the exertion and evaluate the ratings in controlled situations that are as similar as possible to the exercise situations at home. In this way each person can be rather well "calibrated."

In some performances, such as when testing clinical patients, pain may influence a given rating, even at a light or moderate intensity. A specific notation should then be made, for example, "Chest RPE with heart pain" or "Leg RPE with knee pain."

## RPE During a Test on the Bicycle Ergometer

Most test leaders and many people who exercise have a good knowledge of the meaning of results from tests on the bicycle ergometer. In this section, some empirical data are presented to facilitate the understanding of RPE responses.

To illustrate how the RPE scale functions, the relationship between ratings of perceived exertion and exercise intensity (power) for work on a bicycle ergometer with a stepwise increase of the power levels and 5 min work per level for normal, healthy men and women about 35 to 40 years of age are shown in figure 7.2, $a$ and $b$. In the figure the lower line represents subjects with good aerobic fitness, about two standard deviations below the mean (the middle line); the upper line represents those who are less fit, about two standard deviations above the mean. The total area between the outer lines includes about 95% of the subjects. Figure 7.2 can show only the approximate relationship between RPE and power, since the absolute levels depend on the fitness of the groups tested, test conditions, and other factors. A similar relationship is found for running on a treadmill when the stimulus intensity is measured from 1 to 10 mph.

The dispersion in the groups mentioned in the preceding paragraph is about 10% of the RPE. This is also the case for HR. However, a competitive athlete may be able to bike at 300 W, whereas a sick person may manage only 50 W or less.

If the purpose of the exercise test is to make a rough estimate of a person's physical working capacity or to study physiological symptoms of clinical interest, the test is usually stopped at a HR of 170 or 150 beats/min for people about 30 to 50 years old. This HR corresponds roughly to an RPE rating of 15 to 17. For people about 50 to 70 years of age, the test is often stopped at a HR of 150 or 130 beats/min, and for older people still lower. These HRs also correspond to an RPE rating of 15 to 17. Depending on the fitness, age, and health of the subject, the test may have to be

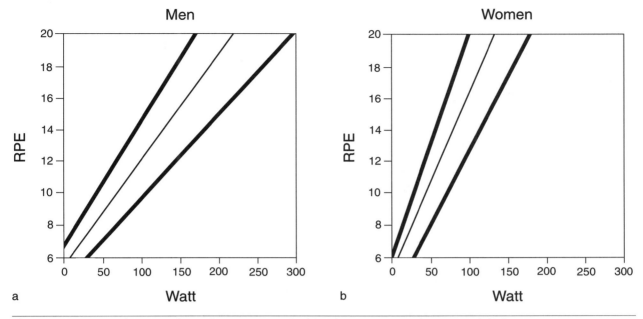

**Figure 7.2** RPE as a function of exercise (power) on the bicycle ergometer (*a*) for men and (*b*) for women.

stopped much sooner due to clinical signs and symptoms.

The relationship between RPE and HR for work done on a bicycle ergometer using the methods described in the preceding paragraphs is shown in figure 7.3 for both men and women. The middle curve is the mean and the two outer lines indicate about two standard deviations above and below the mean.

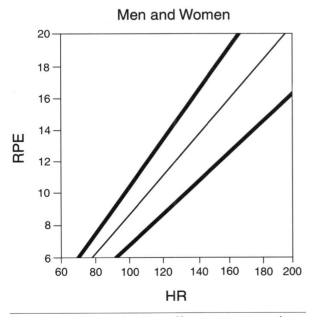

**Figure 7.3** RPE as a function of heart rate (HR) on the bicycle ergometer for both men and women.

# The Borg CR10 Scale

The administration of the CR10 scale should first follow the general principles given at the beginning of this chapter for the RPE scale. Since the Borg CR10 scale (see figure 7.4) is a general intensity scale constructed according to special category-ratio principles, the instructions should, however, be more detailed. Preferably, simple examples should also be given to check that the subject has understood the scale and how to use it. In addition, a special complementary instruction for the modality to be tested (e.g., perceived exertion, aches, and pain) must be given. The CR10 scale has also been used for taste, loudness, color, feeling of satisfaction (e.g., in anorectic patients), and other attributes. It has a great potential for testing not only sensory perceptions, but also attributes of a more complex character, such as well-being, discomfort, beauty and utility, and difficulty of daily performances related to risk assessments.

When instructing the subject, the test leader must first explain the scale, show its functions, and describe how it should be used, and then give specific instruction for the modality or attribute to be tested. Both the general and specific instructions that follow are long and detailed. They are provided here so the test leader can gain a good understanding of the administration and, when

# General Instructions for Using the Borg CR10 Scale

You will use this scale to tell how strong your perception of a certain attribute is. As you can see, the scale stretches from "nothing at all" to "absolute maximum." "Extremely strong—max P" (10) is such an extremely strong perception of a certain attribute that it is the strongest one you have ever experienced: "max P." It may, however, be possible to experience or to imagine a magnitude that is even stronger than what you yourself have previously experienced. Therefore, "absolute maximum", the "highest possible" level, is placed somewhat farther down the scale without a fixed number and marked with a "•". If you should perceive an intensity to be stronger than 10, "extremely strong—max P," you may use numbers on the scale above 10, such as 11, 12, or even higher. "Extremely weak," corresponding to 0.5 on the scale, is something just noticeable, i.e., something that is on the boundary of what is possible to perceive.

You use the scale in the following way: Always start by *looking at the verbal expressions*. Then choose a *number*. If your perception corresponds to "very weak," you say 1. If it is "moderate," you say 3, and so on. You may use whatever numbers you want, also half values, such as 1.5 or 2.5, or decimals, e.g., 0.3, 0.8, 1.7, 2.3, 5.6, or 11.5. It is very important that you answer what *you* perceive and not what you believe you ought to answer. Be as *honest* as possible and try not to overestimate or underestimate the intensities. Remember to start by looking at the verbal expressions before every rating, then give a number.

| | | |
|---|---|---|
| 0 | Nothing at all | "No P" |
| 0.3 | | |
| 0.5 | Extrememly weak | Just noticeable |
| 1 | Very weak | |
| 1.5 | | |
| 2 | Weak | Light |
| 2.5 | | |
| 3 | Moderate | |
| 4 | | |
| 5 | Strong | Heavy |
| 6 | | |
| 7 | Very strong | |
| 8 | | |
| 9 | | |
| 10 | Extremely strong | "Max P" |
| 11 | | |
| ⤢ | | |
| ● | Absolute maximum | Highest possible |

Borg CR10 scale
© Gunnar Borg, 1981, 1982, 1998

Any questions?

*Some examples of items to rate.* The test leader may want to use some simple items for training and testing the subject's rating behavior, and ask the following questions:

To see that you have understood the instruction and how to use the scale, please answer the following questions:

1. How black do you perceive a piece of pure black charcoal to be? (9) How white? (0.5)
2. How loud do you perceive an ordinary conversation between two people to be? (2.5)
3. How white do you perceive a piece of pure white sugar to be? (9) How black? (0.5)
4. How sour do you perceive a lemon to be? (7)
5. How sweet is a ripe banana? (3.5)

The answers to these questions are given in approximate numbers.
Any further questions?

# Complementary Instruction for Perceived Exertion Using the Borg CR10 Scale

We want you to rate your perception of exertion, that is, how heavy and strenuous the exercise feels to you. The perception of exertion depends mainly on the strain and fatigue in your muscles and on your feeling of breathlessness or aches in the chest.

We want you to use this scale from 0 to 10 and "•", where 0 means "no exertion at all" and 10 means "extremely strong—max P", that is, the maximal exertion you have previously experienced.

**1**    corresponds to "very light" exercise. For a normal, healthy person it is like walking slowly at his or her own pace for several minutes.

**3**    on the scale is "moderate" exercise, it is not especially hard, it feels fine, and it is no problem to continue exercising.

**5**    corresponds to "heavy" exercise; it feels hard and you are tired, but you don't have any great difficulties in going on.

**7**    is "very hard" and very strenuous. A healthy person can still go on but he or she has to push him- or herself a lot. It feels very heavy and the person is very tired.

**10**    on the scale is an extremely strenuous exercise level. It is "max P." For most people this is an exercise as strenuous as they have ever experienced before in their lives.

**•**    The dot denotes a perceived exertion that is stronger than 10, "extremely strong." It is your "absolute maximum," for example, 12, 13, or even higher. It is the highest possible level of exertion.

Try to appraise your feeling of exertion as honestly as possible, without thinking about what the actual physical load is. Don't underestimate it, but don't overestimate it either. It's your own feeling of effort and exertion that's important, not how it compares to other people's. What other people think is not important either. Look at the scale and the expressions and then give a number.

What "max exertion"—your "max P"—have you previously experienced in your life? Use that as "10". Any further questions?

necessary, can complement the shorter instructions to the subjects printed on the back of the scales in the appendix.

The administration of the scale should also include specific instructions for each modality being tested. When the Borg CR10 scale is used to test perceived exertion, most of the same principles previously presented for using the RPE scale should be considered.

To be able to compare RPE values obtained with the Borg RPE scale and those obtained with the Borg CR10 scale, a transformation table has been worked out. Table 7.1 shows how CR values (RPE according to the CR10 scale) are obtained from given RPE values according to the RPE scale. The transformation table can also be used for rough transformations in the other direction from the CR10 scale to the RPE scale (Borg and Ottoson 1986).

**Table 7.1.** Scale Transformation

| RPE scale | CR10 scale |
|---|---|
| 6 | 0.0 |
| 7 | 0.0 |
| 8 | 0.5 |
| 9 | 1.0 |
| 10 | 1.5 |
| 11 | 2.0 |
| 12 | 3.0 |
| 13 | 3.5 |
| 14 | 4.5 |
| 15 | 5.5 |
| 16 | 6.5 |
| 17 | 7.5 |
| 18 | 9.0 |
| 19 | 10.0 |
| 20 | 12.0 |

Higher CR10 values than 12 are seldom obtained. In most applied situations with healthy subjects perceiving normal exertion without extreme pain or breathing difficulties, no ratings above 12 need to be registered by the test leader.

## Determining Pain Intensities With the Borg CR10 Scale

When scaling pain with the CR10 scale, the general administration principles previously given for scaling perceived exertion should, of course, also be followed. It is also necessary to follow the general instructions for the CR10 scale, which should be given for all modalities tested. In addition, specific instructions for scaling pain should be given. Since there are many different kinds of pain—in different parts of the body, from different injuries, and so on—it is important to ask the person about the qualities of pain that he or she has at the moment. The person should also tell about previous experiences of pain and try to evaluate the different kinds of pain and their intensities in relation to a certain previous pain or a certain perceived exertion. If a patient comes to a clinic for a certain back pain, and has had previous experiences of similar pain, the conception of that pain can be used as an anchor.

## Specific Instructions When Scaling Pain With the Borg CR10 Scale

Tell me the three worst experiences of pain you have ever had.

If you use 10 as the heaviest physical effort and exertion you have ever experienced or can think of, how strong would you say that your three different pain experiences have been?

$$P_1 =$$

$$P_2 =$$

$$P_3 =$$

Number 10 on the scale, "extremely strong—max P," will now be anchored in your previously experienced worst pain, that is, the worst of the pain you just described. It will now be called "max P."

The worst pain that you have experienced, the "max P," may not be the highest possible level of pain. There may be a level of pain that is still worse than your own "max P." If that feeling of pain is somewhat stronger, for example, 10% stronger than your 10, you will say 11. If it is 20% stronger, you will say 12, and if it is much stronger, e.g., 50% stronger or 1.5 times as strong as your 10, "max P," you will say 15!

Any questions?

It is important to have a good protocol and make notations of all responses, questions, and answers, as well as behavioral or physical reactions.

When interpreting a pain response, remember that its magnitude is often influenced by emotional factors (e.g., the suffering of the individual) and by cognitive and motivational factors (see chapter 9). Seldomly pain ratings above 20 are reasonable and, except for extremely special cases, no values above 20 may be registered. Most often it is the intraindividual level and variation that is of interest and that is most often possible to evaluate using the spontaneous, directly given responses. However, the memories of pain that form the basis for the conceived magnitudes may be rather misleading. Interindividual comparisons are therefore often of doubtful value.

# PART III

# Applications of the Scaling Methods

# Chapter 8

## Perceived Exertion in Working Capacity Tests

There are many tests used to evaluate physical working capacity. Typically, the power level on the bicycle ergometer (at a constant pedaling rate) or the slope and speed on the treadmill are increased in steps, with a specific duration of exercise at each level (see figure 8.1).

The aerobic work capacity—the capacity of the body to do heavy work with large muscle groups lasting several minutes—is commonly defined and measured as an individual's maximal oxygen uptake ($\dot{V}O_2max$). The maximal intensity ($W_{max}$) at which an individual can exercise for a specified time (e.g., 5 min) gives a measurement of the aerobic working capacity that is highly correlated with $\dot{V}O_2max$. The anaerobic capacity—the capacity to do heavy work without oxygen consumption—is often measured with a short-term (e.g., 30 s) maximal performance on a bicycle ergometer. In both the aerobic and anaerobic tests RPE is a useful test variable.

## Aerobic Exercise Testing and RPE

During an aerobic test a subject is usually asked to rate his or her perceived exertion (overall RPE) toward the end of each workload. He or she may also be asked to specify different symptoms (e.g., chest RPE and local muscle RPE). If the test is not used mainly to estimate working capacity but to provoke signs and symptoms of clinical interest (a clinical stress test), it is interesting to obtain ratings referring predominantly to three different aspects of perceived exertion: breathlessness, chest pain, and exertion and aches from the exercising muscles. A profile of these main symptoms is of special interest for differential diagnoses (see figure 8.2).

In some exercise tests the workload (W) may be regulated so that the power increase is changed depending on the reactions relative to each individual's aerobic capacity. Indicators of the degree of strain during the test are obtained from physiological responses (such as HR) but also from RPE. The rigid time-workload schedule can

| Work load | Time or no. of repetitions | | | | |
|-----------|------|------|------|---|------|
|           | $t_1$ | $t_2$ | $t_3$ |   | $t_n$ |
| $W_1$     |      |      |      |   |      |
| $W_2$     |      |      |      |   |      |
| $W_3$     |      |      |      |   |      |
|           |      |      |      |   |      |
| $W_n$     |      |      |      |   |      |

**Figure 8.1** A matrix showing the change in workload (W) with time (t) in ordinary protocols when testing aerobic capacity, muscular strength, or pain.

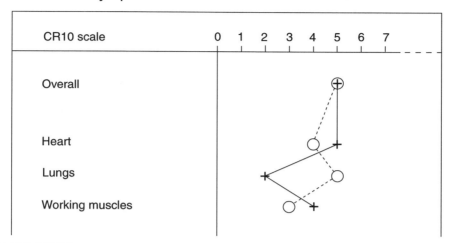

**Figure 8.2** The profile of subjective symptoms may differ between individuals with the same overall perceived exertion, depending on sensations from the heart, lungs, and working muscles.

then be replaced by a more flexible system, evolving directly from the strain and indirectly related to the maximal working capacity of the subject (Borg 1974b).

When it is not necessary to measure the working capacity exactly or when the individual does not want to stress him- or herself or should not do so for medical reasons, a submaximal working capacity can be estimated from the registered HR for a certain high, but not maximal, intensity obtained during a steady-state exercise (according to the Åstrand-Åstrand nomogram, see I. Åstrand 1960; see also P.-O. Åstrand and Rodahl 1986) or from other submaximal tests. From the relationship between HR and W, a linear interpolation or extrapolation can be charted to a certain fixed reference level in HR (to obtain a $W_{HR}$ measurement), for example 170 or 150 bpm (130 bpm for older subjects). The estimated working capacity—for example, $W_{170}$ according to Sjöstrand (1947)—has a high correlation with the actually measured working capacity ($\dot{V}O_2$max or $W_{max}$). In a similar way the working capacity may be estimated from the RPE-W diagram. If a person is exercising at about 80% of his or her working capacity, he or she will usually rate the exertion 17 ("very hard") on the RPE scale. The working capacity thus estimated is often denoted $W_{R17}$ when the W is expressed in watts or $V_{R17}$ when the velocity (V) is the independent variable during the test.

In several experiments the $W_R$ measurement has proven to be highly reliable and valid (Borg 1962a; Borg and Linderholm 1970; Edgren et al.

1976). The reproducibility estimated from intratest correlations is about as good for the $W_R$ measurements as for the $W_{HR}$ measurements.

A study by Borg and Linderholm (1970) calculated the reliability of $W_{R13}$ by correlating two different $W_{R13}$ values obtained from one test. (RPE responses from every second workload were used during a work test with a stepwise increase every sixth minute: 50 W and 150 W for one $W_{R13}$ value, and 100 W and 200 W for another $W_{R13}$ value; both were estimates of working capacity.) The correlation between the two $W_{R13}$ values was high, $r_{xy} = .85$. A reliability coefficient of .92 was then estimated after correction according to Spearman-Brown's split-half formula since a $W_{R13}$ value calculated from all four workloads should be more reliable.

The intratest correlations indicate a low methodological error that tends to decrease with increase in the reference level of HR or RPE. Therefore the reliability (intratest correlation) for $W_{R17}$ should be at least .90. The obtained $W_{170}$ and $W_{R17}$ were both about 200 ± 33 watts (mean ± SD). The error of a single determination ($s_e$) according to the formula

$$s_e = s_x \sqrt{1 - r_{tt}}$$

(where $s_x$ is the standard deviation in the group) should be

$$s_x = 33\sqrt{1 - 0.9} \approx 10 \; W$$

that is, about 5% of the mean value.

The error of the W measures can also be estimated from *repeated examinations* of the same individuals. Using this approach the overall error was estimated from double determinations made with a time interval of 2 to 4 wk (Borg and Linderholm 1970). We chose a comparatively long period between the tests to minimize the effect of memory on the rating of perceived exertion. The measurements based on observations made using relatively high workloads, $W_{170}$ and $W_{R17}$, had a smaller error than those based on observations obtained at relatively low workloads. The error of the determination of the W measures was 5% to 8%.

High validity has been obtained for $W_{R17}$ measures in several studies when actual measurements of working capacity for various daily work or sport performances were used as a criterion. A study with lumber workers (in which the old 21-grade scale was used) used wages from piecerate work, and another study used results from a skiing competition (Borg 1962a). Edgren and coworkers (1976) used results from cross-country runs for validation, as well as results from other physiological and performance tests. Each of these studies obtained correlations between .50 and .70.

Predictions of maximal performances on the bicycle ergometer have been shown to be as good from RPE values as from HR (Morgan and Borg 1977). Since maximal HR decreases with age in about the same way as $\dot{V}O_2max$, but maximal RPE generally does not decrease for healthy subjects who can make a voluntary maximal performance, a certain RPE value is a better reference value than a certain HR. This is especially important in age-heterogeneous populations (Borg and Linderholm 1970; Bar-Or 1977; see also Borg 1978). To increase the validity of $W_{HR}$ measurements and to obtain values comparable with $W_R$, relative HR (RHR, also called HR reserve) should be used:

$$RHR = \frac{HR_x - HR_{rest}}{HR_{max} - HR_{rest}} \times 100$$

where the reference value is corrected according to the range of HR from rest to maximum. In figure 8.3 three different measurements of working capacity based on submaximal HR ($W_{130}$), RPE ($W_{R13}$), and 80% of relative HR ($W_{p80}$) are compared with $\dot{V}O_2max$. As the figure shows, $W_{R13}$ declines with age in a way similar to $\dot{V}O_2max$ and $W_{p80}$.

The term *stress test* is sometimes used for a test of working capacity if the main aim is "stressing" patients to provoke important signs and symptoms that are not found at rest, as previously

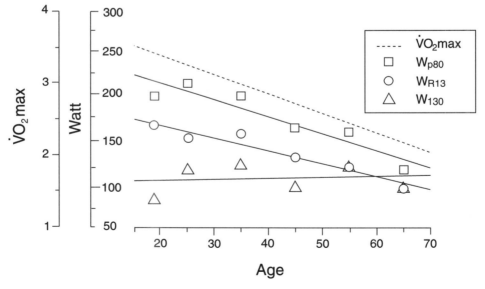

**Figure 8.3**  Change in physical working capacity with age. The top dashed line shows the decline of $\dot{V}O_2max$ (from Åstrand and Rodahl 1986). The next three solid lines show estimates of aerobic capacity based on submaximal tests (from Borg and Linderholm 1970). The uppermost of the solid lines shows estimates of aerobic capacity according to $W_{p80}$, the workload at which the subject can work at 80% of his or her HR range. The next line shows the variation of the $W_{R13}$ measurements, the workload at which the subject gives an RPE of "somewhat hard." The lowest line shows the variation of $W_{130}$ measurements, the workload at which the subject has a HR of 130 bpm.

described. A clinician must use more precautions when stressing a patient so that the test can be interrupted quickly if there are severe signs or symptoms. It is important to have a proper warm-up period and use small increases of the workload. The clinician should record ECG and other physiological measurements during a stress test, depending on the physical condition of the test subject, and subjective symptoms also. The test is often performed according to a predetermined, rigid schedule, and the patient has to exercise at gradually increasing intensity levels. Often the duration of exercise at each level is 2 to 5 min. Sometimes the exercise is continuous, and sometimes it increases by steps every minute. To obtain reliable and valid ratings, the patient should exercise at least 2 min (preferably 3 or 4) at each load because two to three ratings are often desirable: breathlessness, chest (heart) pain (or just chest exertion, including breathlessness and pain), and exertion from the main peripheral muscles and joints involved in the exercise.

As previously mentioned, monitoring RPE during a stress test is important to facilitate the decision of when to interrupt the test for safety reasons, especially for patients and elderly people. Continue the test until there are physiological signs of dangerous strain or until the ratings are higher than appropriate for the physical exercise. A rough rule adopted by several clinics is to interrupt the test at RPE 14 to 15 (or 5 on the Borg CR10 scale). Remember, when it's "hard," it's too hard! In healthy subjects and young athletes RPE 17 (or CR10 7) is a better level for interruption since this higher level gives a more valid estimate of working capacity.

# Anaerobic Exercise Testing and RPE

As discussed in the preceding section, RPE is often used in ergometer tests designed to evaluate aerobic working capacity. There is an increasing interest in anaerobic tests, however. The Wingate test (see Bar-Or 1987) is an example of a short-term (30 s) maximal exercise test in which subjects pedal at a maximal frequency against a resistance set relative to their body weight. Bar-Or has shown the test to be reliable and valid.

In short-term maximal performance tests it is difficult to set a resistance that is optimal for each individual. Since the anaerobic capacity is not known before the test, the question is: What resistance will lead to exhaustion after precisely the desired time (e.g., 30 s)?

## Cycling Strength Test

The first anaerobic bicycle ergometer test to measure dynamic muscular strength was my Cycling Strength Test (CST; Borg 1961a, 1962a). In this test the pedal resistance is increased linearly with time during exercise until the subject cannot maintain the stipulated pedaling rate. CST determinations are usually performed on a special electrically braked bicycle ergometer, where resistance is not affected by changes in the pedaling rate. The power increase is set, for example, to 8 W / s and the pedaling rate (r) to 60 rpm. One CST assessment ordinarily takes 40 to 50 s, of which only the last 10 s involve very hard exercise.

Perceived exertion may be used to facilitate the construction of a short-term test in which the individual exercises at a constant speed and a constant resistance suitably adapted for him or her. A great difficulty with this, however, is identifying the appropriate resistance for the subject. Since performance time becomes the dependent variable and depends on the chosen resistance and the capacity of the subject tested, it is difficult to control time as an independent variable. In the Wingate test the resistance is kept constant, but the pedaling speed is not, and in the CST the speed is kept constant, but the resistance is not. To keep both speed and resistance constant is practically impossible if we do not know in advance the capacity of the subject to be tested. To solve this problem we need to know both the approximate capacity of the individual tested and the equation that gives the relation between resistance (W) and performance time (T). If we know these factors, we can utilize the general equation for predictions in individual cases.

The capacity to work maximally at a certain power level for a short period of time (e.g., 0.5 min) can be predicted fairly well from RPE values and from HR. In a submaximal, incremental test (comprising 0.5 min work and 0.5 min rest, i.e., a stepwise increase every minute) a combination of these indicators seems to give the best prediction (where 80% of the age-corrected $HR_{max}$ is used as a reference value for 0.5 min maximal performance and a corresponding RPE value of 20; Borg 1982b). This prediction of $W_{max0.5}$—that is, the mean value of the two estimated predictors: $W_{max0.5} = 1/2\ (W_{0.5HR} + W_{0.5RPE})$—can be used together with the general function in a new CST with constant load (CST-C).

The equation describing the general relation between W and T for this kind of exercise relies on experiments by Grosse-Lordemann and Müller (1937), Tornvall (1963), and Borg and Nordheden (1976). The equation is $T = c \times W^n$, where the exponent $n \cong -4$. The variation of log T with log W is described in figure 8.4.

## CST-C

In a first CST-C assessment the subjects pedal at the estimated level (according to the prediction based on the submaximal test described in the preceding section) for as long as possible. The performance time is measured and used to correct the power level according to the equation (figure 8.4). After a rest of 5 min a second assessment is carried out on the corrected power level. The subject then pedals at close to the desired 30-s power level, and after a new correction a final CST-C-measurement is obtained.

Two different studies have obtained high reliability coefficients (estimated from correlations between assessments): $r_{xy} = .96$ to .98. The results have also been correlated with measurements from the old CST and the Wingate test (Borg, unpublished reports). The correlation obtained with the old CST was high ($r_{xy} = .90$) and also fairly high with the Wingate test ($r_{xy} = .70$ to .90).

# Estimating Maximal and Resting Heart Rates

To evaluate the importance of heart rate (HR) as a measure of exercise intensity, it is necessary to know a subject's maximal and resting HR values. However, because of practical or medical reasons, it is often not possible to measure maximal HR; thus estimates are made from age-related norms. These estimates are, however, very rough since people differ in maximal HR both when they are young and in how it regresses with age.

One method of estimation tried in some investigations (see Borg 1977; Wilmore et al. 1986) uses the relationship between RPE and HR to predict maximal HR. We know that during a bicycle ergometer test, for example, there is a linear increase in both RPE and HR and that when people have to exercise for several minutes to reach maximum, they usually rate perceived exertion at about 19. Since the RPE scale has a built-in maximal value, this value can be used to predict maximal HR. A submaximal test with stepwise increase of the power levels is used, and both HR and RPE are recorded. The method is described in figure 8.5.

In the diagram RPE is used as the independent variable and maximal HR is predicted from submaximal measurements by extrapolation to a certain predetermined level of reference (e.g., RPE 19). This method has been found to function well but seems to depend greatly on good instruction and competent subjects.

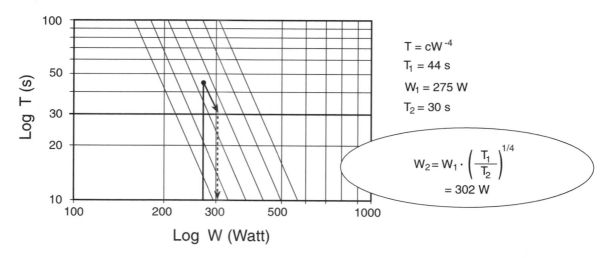

$$T = cW^{-4}$$
$$T_1 = 44\ s$$
$$W_1 = 275\ W$$
$$T_2 = 30\ s$$

$$W_2 = W_1 \cdot \left(\frac{T_1}{T_2}\right)^{1/4}$$
$$= 302\ W$$

**Figure 8.4**  The general relationship between resistance (power, W, in watts) and performance time (T, in seconds) and how an obtained result may be corrected to the desired 30-s level.

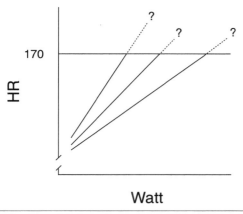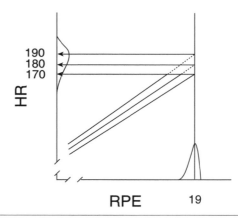

**Figure 8.5** A model showing how to estimate HR$_{max}$ from the HR-RPE diagram. The model may also be used to estimate HR at rest (and may also be applied to other variables).

One can similarly determine resting HR. Because some individuals' HRs are elevated before a test due to pretest activities, anxiety in the test situation, or a more stable elevation because of an acute infection or a pathological state, a measurement of resting HR at this time is often misleading. To estimate resting HR from RPE (or the relationship between HR and power), an extrapolation may be made to RPE 6, or a zero power level (see figure 8.6).

# The Simple Run or Walk Test

The interest in physical training and exercise creates a need for individuals to be able to determine their own fitness and aerobic capacity at

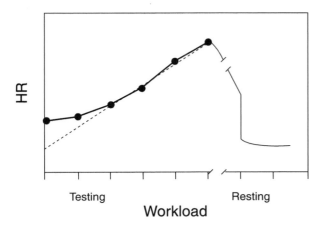

**Figure 8.6** A schematic figure showing the change in HR (bpm) with workload (power in watt and time in min.) during an exercise test with subjects with initial test anxiety.

regular intervals. Tests of working capacity are common for diagnosing cardiopulmonary diseases or for athletes but are uncommon for other individuals interested in monitoring changes in physical fitness using easily assessable, reliable, and valid test results.

Ergometers enable good measurements of working capacity but unfortunately are rather expensive. For this reason several simple, inexpensive tests have been designed that can be performed without any special ergometers but that still satisfy the demands for a good test. For the ordinary person one such test is the simple walk or run test, which we have developed and which we hope turns out to be a meaningful contribution to the existing arsenal of methods (Borg 1970a, 1970b; Borg, Edgren, and Marklund 1971, 1973; Borg and Ohlsson 1975).

In the design of a simple test, some key demands must be met:

1. It should be risk-free and easy for the individual to administer.

2. It should not call for expensive apparatuses.

3. It should stimulate the interest of the individual.

4. It should be reliable and valid.

5. It is an advantage if the test can be tied in with everyday, natural activities, such as walking or running, and can be done both indoors and in the open air.

A safe test situation implies moderate exercise intensities and activities chosen from everyday life, where the technique to perform is well learned and does not cause great variation in the results. The exercise period should be short

---

## Can a Subjective Variable Be Used as an "Independent Variable"?

Some of my best research ideas have come to me during light jogging, walking, or traveling by train. One nice autumn day at the end of the 1960s, after taking part in a sport science conference during which my ideas of using subjective variables in testing and training were challenged by some physiologists, I took a long walk to the railroad station. These challenges to my ideas had provoked a strong defensive reaction, and I came up with all kinds of applications for subjective evaluation systems.

We had started studies using perceived exertion in monitoring exercise intensity. Some experiments indicated that when keeping a constant speed while running, perceived exertion for rather hard exercise increases somewhat. HR may arrive at a steady state, but perceived exertion increases over time. On this walk I realized that to maintain perceived exertion, running speed possibly must decrease slowly. I decided it might be possible to combine perceived exertion with perception of speed using perceived exertion as the main cue. (A certain running speed doesn't tell us how hard it is. Even a very slow speed may be hard for some.) A second thought was to use the conception and the perception of speed to monitor exercise intensity during a simple run test. While sitting and relaxing on the train, I then constructed a simple run (or walk) test as a home test using a subjective variable (the perceived speed) as the "independent variable" instead of objective speed.

---

enough to motivate people to complete the test, but long enough to involve circulatory adaptation so that the test indicates aerobic working capacity.

If the test is designed as a walk test, the speed of walking should not be too low because during a low effort HR is not especially reliable and the relationship between HR and speed is not linear (Böje 1944; Borg 1973b; Borg et al. 1987). During running, higher and more valid values are obtained, which means that running may be preferable to walking. However, if the running test is designed as a maximal test, it will be difficult for the test subjects to follow the instruction to maintain a constant speed, which is a necessary ground for the validity of the test.

In a submaximal treadmill test of aerobic capacity, the individual has to walk or run at different slopes or velocities that vary from low to high continuously or, more commonly, in steps, with one or a few minutes exercise at each intensity level. In a typical situation the test leader controls and varies the intensity (e.g., the speed) as the independent variable. HR, $VO_2$max, blood lactate, or other physiological responses and RPE (overall, central, or local) are the dependent variables. A common way to then estimate the working capacity is to plot HR against speed, slope, or speed-slope combination, depending on the protocol, and to determine the speed at a given reference value in HR (e.g., 170 or 150 bpm) from the HR diagram by interpolation or extrapolation.

For a walk or run test an even track of the right length should be used in order to strain the circulatory organs to such an extent that a steady-state level can be reached (i.e., about 5 min or more; Åstrand and Saltin 1961). For a walk test by a group of people who are untrained, elderly, or medical patients, a 400-m (or quarter-mile) track or just around the block at home can be adequate. For a run test the distance should be about twice as long (800 m or half a mile). To test physically fit persons who are accustomed to prolonged endurance training, the distance should be longer (e.g., 1,600 m or one mile).

It is important that a person can test him- or herself properly without the help of an instructor. When outside the laboratory walking on a track, a person cannot control the velocity as the independent variable in a physical way, as can be done on a treadmill. It is, however, possible for the individual to control it subjectively if the exercise is not too light or too hard. Most people have no trouble walking (or jogging slowly) at a constant speed. If they are doing so, they are performing well-defined work, carrying their own bodies for a certain duration or distance. Studies by Borg, Edgren, and Marklund (1971) and by Edgren and Borg (1975) have shown that it is possible to make stable performances at slightly different speeds with a high degree of reliability according to given instructions (e.g., "Run slowly at your own preferred and constant speed"). The given distance (e.g., half a mile) is then an independent variable. The time used to cover the given distance is determined as a dependent variable, together with HR or RPE. The speed is then calculated from the time and used as an independent variable.

No technical apparatus is used to regulate the speed; it is determined solely by the instruction given, the test subject's understanding of the instruction, and his or her perception of speed and exertion. When the subject has covered a given distance, the time, HR, and RPE are recorded. In this manner a measure of the person's achievement and the "cost" behind the achievement are obtained.

After a short (1-min) rest the person repeats the exercise. This can be done several more times with variations in the instruction; for instance, the subject is told the first time to "run very slowly and at a constant speed" and the second time to "run somewhat faster than before but still in a calm tempo and at a constant speed." For a possible third repetition the individual can be told to "run somewhat faster still—that is, rather fast—without exerting maximum effort but continuing to maintain a constant speed." If two determinations are carried out, two points are obtained in a diagram in which speed (in m/s or yd/s) is plotted on the $x$-axis and the HR (or RPE) is plotted on the $y$-axis. A physical fitness value can then be calculated in the form of the velocity at a given reference level in HR (or RPE), for example, 150 bpm (RPE 15), 170 bpm, or for elderly people, 130 bpm (see figure 8.7). For a walk test choose a reference level about 30 bpm lower.

The linearity among HR, RPE, and running velocity is good within a limited speed range. If the general growth function of HR in relation to

velocity is known for the test subject in question or for people similar to the test subject, it is sufficient to determine one point in the diagram empirically, that is, one velocity value with a corresponding HR (or RPE). An extrapolation can then be made to the reference level using knowledge of the general slope of the HR (or RPE)–velocity function.

The reliability and validity of the simple run test were studied in an experiment by Borg and Ohlsson (1975). Twenty-five men about 19 years old were tested on three different occasions. For the first test they had to run 800 m three times with a 1-min rest between repetitions. After a 30-min rest they ran 1,200 m two times, also with a 1-min rest between repetitions. On the second test occasion each person individually ran 1,500 m at his voluntary maximal speed. The time for 1,500 m was used as a test criterion. On the third test occasion a bicycle ergometer test was performed as a second criterion.

A test reliability coefficient was determined by correlating the results from the different runs. High correlations were obtained for the $V_{170}$: .91 and .97 for the successive 800-m runs and .94 for the 1,200-m run. The validity coefficients in the form of correlations with the 1,500-m run were all high: between .58 and .70 for 800 m and for 1,200 m. The correlations with the submaximal estimates of working capacity from the bicycle ergometer test were high (.60 to .76), both when calculated from RPE ($W_{R17}$) and from HR ($W_{170}$). There was no gain in validity in extending the distance from 800 m to 1,200 m, nor in running three times instead of two. Subsequent studies (Borg, Herbert, and Ceci 1984) have cross-validated the high reliability and validity coefficients and found them to be about the same. RPE may be used instead of HR, but most often HR is preferred and perceived exertion is instead commonly used to help the subject check the exercise intensity during running.

The test is mainly intended as a method to compare changes in each individual's fitness (in running capacity). Only very rough comparisons with other individuals can be made. In our Swedish studies on young men (15 to 35 years old) a mean value in $V_{170}$ around 3.5 m/s was obtained, with a standard deviation of about 0.7 m/s. The average result in $V_{170}$, covering about 50% of these men, was between 3.0 and 4.0. The very best runners had values above 5.0, and the worst below 2.0. A comparable group of women (see Hassmén and Ceci 1990) had $V_{170}$ results about 10% lower.

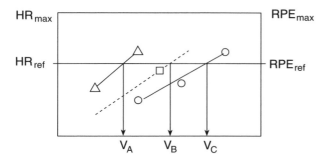

**Figure 8.7**  The principle behind the simple run test with obtained HR (or RPE) plotted against obtained speed (V). A submaximal reference level (HR_ref or RPE_ref) is chosen for estimating working capacity for three different individuals (A, B, and C).

For a walk test, both reliability and validity coefficients are slightly lower. They are, however, good enough for practical use. Moreover, for patients or elderly subjects the walk test is a good alternative to the run test. It is essential that the subjects use an ordinary walking technique but still try to walk as economically as possible. (If they want to be able to compare themselves with other people, the technique may be more essential for walking than for running). The test should be used primarily as an individual test with intraindividual comparisons on different occasions (e.g., in connection with rehabilitation, weight loss, or training programs).

The same principles used for the run or walk test can also be used in other kinds of exercise (e.g., in swimming, bicycling, or cross-country skiing). The weather conditions, wind, temperature, and surface of the track may greatly influence the results. For each individual who wants to test him- or herself, this does not matter much as long as the conditions and the technique used are similar on the different test occasions.

# Chapter 9

## Scaling Pain and Related Subjective Somatic Symptoms

As mentioned in chapter 8, the primary purpose of clinical ergometer tests of patients is not to obtain an exact measure of working capacity, but to stress the patient to provoke signs and symptoms of diagnostic value, such as objective physiological responses (including ECG patterns) and subjective responses (such as aches and pains in the legs, joints, or chest). Subjects may experience breathlessness (dyspnea), headaches, dizziness, feelings of heat, stomach problems (feeling sick), or specific heart pains. If one special symptom is more intense than the others, it dominates the pattern and may be of special clinical importance. Furthermore, subjects may feel fear and anxiety related to their health condition. Notations about these kinds of subjective symptoms are commonly made during clinical exercise tests, pointing to the need for a simple, standardized method for quantitative assessment of some main subjective symptoms.

## Evaluating Symptoms and Pain

Borg, Karlsson, and Lindblad (1976) carried out the first extensive study on several subjective somatic symptoms. The experiment aimed to study changes in certain subjective symptoms in normal people during prolonged exercise with increasing workload and the relationship of these changes to HR. Thirty-two healthy subjects performed physical exercise on a bicycle ergometer.

Workloads of 20, 40, 60, and 100 W were used during working periods of 6 min each. After 100 W the increase was 50 W every sixth minute until the subjects reached a HR of 170 bpm or rated 17 on the RPE scale.

At the end of each 6-min period each subject estimated perceived intensity in terms of perceived exertion, leg fatigue, leg pain, chest pain, panting, and severe breathing difficulties (dyspnea). A 9-grade category scale was used (the new CR10 scale was not yet developed) with numbers from 0 ("Nothing whatsoever") to 8 ("Maximal") and scale steps from 1 ("Very, very weak") to 7 ("Very, very hard"). This scale is rather similar to the RPE scale and linearly related to it, and thus also to power and HR. Subjects used this scale for all symptoms except overall perceived exertion, for which they used the RPE scale.

Somewhat linear relationships were found among HR, RPE, and ratings with the 9-grade scale. Figure 9.1 presents the changes in intensity of each symptom (with ratings transformed to the CR10 scale) and in HR for a very fit group of 16 subjects. These results correspond well with those of another group consisting of 16 less-fit (with regard to relative responses) subjects.

As figure 9.1 shows, perceived exertion, leg fatigue, panting, and HR show a similar trend over workload. There are clear differences between these variables and leg pain, breathing difficulties, and chest pain, which show much lower values and also clear differences in their respective trends. Correlation coefficients were calculated on the results from 100 W and 200 W. Very high correlations were found in the two groups

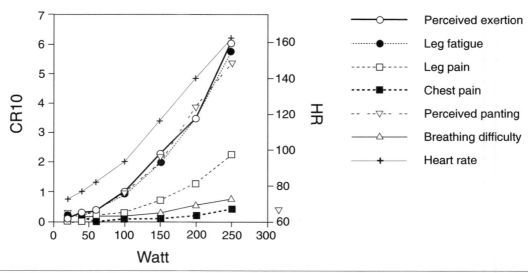

**Figure 9.1** The increase of HR and subjective somatic symptoms (see symbols) according to the Borg CR10 scale with power (in watts) in bicycling in a strong group of healthy males (from Borg, Karlsson, and Lindblad 1976; original ratings translated to CR10 scale).

at both 100 W and 200 W for perceived exertion, leg fatigue, and panting (most correlations being between .60 and .90). In the total group, the correlations were above .90. Therefore, in a healthy group of subjects, good predictions can be made from one of these variables to the others, for example from leg fatigue to normal breathlessness (panting).

The correlation between the two pain variables, leg pain and chest pain, was weak or nonsignificant. The same was true between chest pain and perceived exertion. Leg pain correlated significantly (around .50) with perceived exertion and leg exertion at 100 and 200 W. Breathing difficulty did not correlate with perceived exertion or panting, except in the case of the weakest group of subjects at the highest workload, for whom breathing difficulty correlated with panting ($r_{xy}$ = .55). Breathing difficulty showed a rather high correlation with chest pain, however, especially in the less-fit group of subjects ($r_{xy}$ = .70 and .53 at the two workloads). Therefore, in a total, heterogeneous group of subjects a rather high correlation may be predicted between chest pain and breathing difficulty (dyspnea).

The results of this study by Borg, Karlsson, and Lindblad (1976) are of interest to understand how healthy people function, to understand how their symptoms correlate, and as a reference study for differential diagnostics in patients with cardiovascular or pulmonary disorders. A heightened breathlessness, above that which can be predicted from the exercise intensity according to leg exer-

tion or perception of pedal resistance (in absence of estimates of the individual's working capacity), may thus indicate a pulmonary disorder.

The different symptoms may form a profile in which one or a few symptoms dominate over the others. For example, if three main symptoms recorded are (1) breathlessness, (2) heart pain, and (3) leg exertion, different profiles may be obtained depending on the disease. In patients with angina pectoris the normal and rather linear increase of chest pain may start to increase much more at a certain intensity level. This may also happen to breathlessness or perceived exertion in the legs if cardiopulmonary disease causes pain because of insufficient oxygen supply to the working muscles. Often the test is interrupted by the patient before really severe symptoms are reported (e.g., at 5 on the CR10 scale) because the patient does not have the capacity or motivation to exercise at a higher intensity level. Figure 8.2 in chapter 8 gives an example of a profile of symptoms: overall perceived exertion together with symptoms from the heart, lungs, and working muscles.

Using a 9-grade category scale like the one previously described (Borg, Karlsson, and Lindblad 1976), but with numbers from 1 to 9 to avoid zero, 63 male patients (mean age 54 years) with diagnosed coronary heart disease and severe angina pectoris participated in a study on the development of pain during physical stress (Borg, Holmgren, and Lindblad 1981). All patients performed a bicycle ergometer test; the power began at 10 W and was increased by 10 W every minute. ECG was recorded during the test, and ratings of perceived chest pain were registered at the end of each workload. The patients were instructed to recollect the strongest bout of angina pectoris they had ever experienced and to use that as a frame of reference; this pain level was to be equivalent to "extremely strong," 8 or 9 on the scale. The pain level that forced the patient to stop walking in daily life was used as a second reference; this level was to be equivalent to 5 or 6 on the scale ("not so light, quite strong, strong").

With reference data from our laboratory, the ratings were roughly transformed to the CR10 scale for comparisons. The patients were classified into three groups by length of working time (fairly strong to maximal working capacity). The increase in pain was similar in all three groups after rating 2. In the first group (the group with most severe signs and symptoms) pain began to occur at very light power, and the subsequent increase was fairly linear. The trend was the same in the other two groups, even though the test lasted longer and the patients were able to exercise at higher levels before experiencing pain. The main characteristic of the growth function was a slow increase initially and then rather abruptly a strong increase. In relation to HR, the ratings at heavy loads were higher than might be expected in healthy people according to the study by Borg, Karlsson, and Lindblad (1976). This finding is similar to the previous result from Borg and Linderholm (1970).

# Scaling Pain With the Borg CR10 Scale

For testing patients with musculoskeletal disorders, principles similar to those for an ergometer test can be used. It is as important to recognize and evaluate the subjective symptoms of patients with musculoskeletal disorders as those of cardiopulmonary patients. Back pain, joint pain (especially the knee and the hip), and various muscle pains are very common and do not seem to decrease as expected from improvements in working conditions. Maybe modern civilization also has made humanity more sensitive and vulnerable to these kinds of disorders or more consciously aware of them.

Many different methods of psychophysical scaling have been used to rate pain. The intensity of pain and its variation in a rather simple, sensory dimension has been the focus of experimentally induced pain on healthy subjects with a good understanding of the rather difficult scaling methodology. Common methods taken from psychophysical scaling of most sensory attributes together with specific instructions for pain have been applied (Algom and Lubel 1994; Ellermeier, Westphal, and Heidenfelder 1991; Ahlquist and Franzén 1994; Gracely and Dubner 1981). Methods in clinical cases have to include most of the different qualitative and quantitative aspects of pain with an integration of perceptual, behavioral, and physiological variables. To compare the qualities and levels of diagnostic pain, special reference material is also needed, taking into account the population of individuals, the kind and context of pain, and the purpose of the examination.

Things are simpler in experimental studies of pain than in clinical diagnostics since it is the general or intraindividual variation to a laboratory stimulus that is most interesting. Some ratio scaling methods have been used in these studies, such as magnitude estimation (ME) and cross-modal matching. Other methods used are the Visual Analog Scale (VAS) and finger span methods (see chapter 4), which some researchers argue give measurements on a ratio level, and category methods as the category partitioning (CP) method developed by Heller (see Ellermeier, Westphal, and Heidenfelder 1991). Boivie, Hansson, and Lindblom (1994), Price (1988), and Turk and Melzack (1992) offer reviews of scaling pain.

The category-ratio scaling principles I've introduced (Borg 1973a; 1982a) have been used to study experimental and clinical pain. Gracely developed similar principles of category-ratio scaling specifically for perception of pain (see Gracely et al. 1978). He used verbal pain descriptors to obtain measurements on a ratio scale that could be used to reliably and validly determine measurements of sensory or affective components of pain.

The previously reported studies on angina pain have been continued. In an experimental study by Sylvén et al. (1988) adenosine was ingested in the blood to provoke pain. A very clear dose-response (S-R) relationship was found using the CR10 scale. The pain was judged to be similar in quality to the angina pain. The S-R function could be described very well by a power function with an exponent of 0.6 and with a very high goodness of fit correlation ($r_{xy}$ = .999).

Harms-Ringdahl and co-workers (1983; see also Harms-Ringdahl et al. 1986) assessed experimental discomfort and pain in loaded passive joint structures. The researchers compared the reliability of the method with the VAS and found a high correlation. In addition to general instructions about the aim of the study and what to rate, each subject pretested on using the scale. The subjects were given stimuli solutions with different concentrations of citric acid and had to judge the degree of sourness. In this way the subjects got both information about the study and training in using the CR10 scale. One of the eight subjects was found unsuitable and did not take part in the experiment.

The results from stimulating the elbow joints with a load (torque in newton-meters [N·m] or joules) of 7 N·m for 6 min showed a rather linear increase of the ratings from 1 to 5 during the first 4 min. For the last 2 min (before the test was interrupted) the curve leveled off to about 7. Great variations were found between individuals. After the load was removed, some subjects rated the pain or discomfort higher than at the end of the session. The sensation then slowly decreased. This investigation is a good example of a way to study pain both over time and over load.

Neely (1995) compared several scaling methods, such as ME, CR scaling, VAS, and the German CP method and found that all methods were useful for their special purposes, but the CR scale was better than ME with regard to level determinations and better than VAS and CP with regard to ratio properties. In a study on experimental somatosensory pain (pressure on a finger by cylinder) the CP scale was compared with CR scaling and found to give similar results. The conclusion drawn by Müller, Neely, and Fichtl (1995) was that "both scales proved to be resistant to bias effects and give reliable results."

Studying musculoskeletal pain in patients using the CR10 scale has become rather common in Sweden. In a study of pain after one knee operation, the effects of pain relief using a usual pharmaceutical drug and electrical transcutaneous nerve stimulation (TNS) were compared with each other and a placebo TNS. The CR scale was found useful for the evaluation of the pain relief also in comparison to electromyographic (EMG) measurements (Arvidsson 1985).

Simply because a scale is used to measure pain does not mean that it is a pain scale per se. A general intensity scale, such as the VAS or the CR10 scale, may be used to estimate loudness or sweetness but also intensities of pain. To qualify as a pain scale, the scale has to be defined and anchored for pain ratings using special pain-related explanations. Compare, for instance, a 5-grade (1 to 5) scale that can be used as an ordinal scale to rank food preferences but that can also be used in a different context and with other specifications as an interval scale for grading scholastic attainments. It is not possible to take a scale from one context and use it in a different one without clearly specifying the conditions.

A great problem when scaling pain is that the intensity greatly depends on the qualities of pain, including specific sensory cues; cognitive, affective, and motivational components; and personality states and traits. The pain may also change or fluctuate over time, depending on the social context and factors related to the interaction between the person and the situation.

The focus of pain assessment may be on relationships among intensities of a general character (time courses and S-R functions for somatosensory pain) that are valid for most human beings, disregarding individual differences. Interest may also focus on individual differences in either S-R functions (describing *relative* variation in pain) or individually anchored pain (giving *absolute* levels of intensities).There may also be comparisons of different qualities of pain from different organs or parts or the body. Many different kinds of measurements thus may be needed if the aim is to study the intra- or interindividual variation, the intra- or intermodal variation, or comparisons of *relationships* or *levels* (see chapter 4). Still another aspect is the interdisciplinary comparison of perceptual estimates with physiological responses or psychomotor performances (see Borg 1994b).

Figure 9.2 shows pain curves for three different individuals (or three different qualities for one individual) to illustrate the difficulties in comparing pain intensities over time. The time (T) scale may be graded in seconds, minutes, hours, days, weeks, or months. The pain intensity scale may be anchored intraindividually with comparisons concerning only the time course for each person (the individual being his or her own control, disregarding differences in levels). Sometimes, however, an intersubjective "unit" is needed, meaning that at least some rough interindividual comparisons of intensity levels should be possible. This kind of comparison is the most difficult and should be avoided if possible. The time courses are different for the three individuals in the figure, but the intensity levels may not really be different. For instance, two individuals' pain may decrease a great deal from $T_2$ to $T_4$ and, perhaps after a long therapy,

decrease even more at $T_n$, but the total level difference between the curves may reflect only differences in rating behavior. The differences in time courses may reflect, however, some rather sudden changes in pain intensity as an effect of therapy.

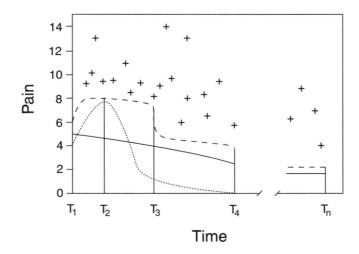

**Figure 9.2** Hypothetical changes of intensities of pain over time. The curves describe overall and mean intensities, while the crosses (+) reflect sudden, very intense "flashes" of pain.

# Chapter 10

# External, Physiological, and Psychological Factors and Perceived Exertion

**M**any factors in the physical and social environment besides the mere exercise-related loads can influence psycho-physiological responses to exertion. In running and cycling there is a simple relationship between RPE and HR. The relationship may vary, however, depending on several interacting conditions of both physical and psychosocial origins. Knowledge about the responses within the effort continua—all the different perceptual, physiological, and performance variables—how they change, and how they interact with each other, is rather limited, however. We know more scientifically about some physiological and performance variables than about perceptual ones. Unfortunately, the understanding of perceptual factors is to a great extent based on folklore or common sense. Much more research is needed.

## The Environment

The physical aspects of the environment include altitude, ambient temperature, music and noise, and air conditions such as wind velocity, humidity, and airborne pollutants. In addition, the social context in which exercise is performed, as it interacts with the physical factors, may have a special influence on the perception of exertion.

When a person exercises in the heat, as when running outdoors on a hot day (e.g., more than 100° F [37.7° C]), the relationship between HR and RPE changes considerably. If the temperature and humidity are very high, as may be the case for firefighters during their work, the relationship may change dramatically, especially if the clothing is not fitted to the task and the person has to work hard or carry heavy loads. HR is then greatly influenced not only by the heavy work, but also by the heat. RPE, on the other hand, is not influenced to the same degree by the heat but more by the actual physical exercise (Gamberale and Holmér 1977).

The conditions shown in figure 10.1 can be both helpful and alarming. It can be good that perceived exertion closely follows the objective exertion related to the actual work stress. There is cause for concern, however, if an athlete or a firefighter underestimates the total strain on the cardiovascular system caused by the combined stress of the exercise and the hot environment. Some people can stand this combination rather well, but others cannot.

How the HR-RPE relationship changes during exercise in a cold environment is not as well known. A slight cooling may have a positive effect on the organism, but a very cold environment is known to be detrimental to performance and may also change the HR-RPE relationship. A good example of this can be seen in athletes cross-country skiing in very cold weather. Breathing may be difficult and cause an increase in RPE that is not followed by an increase in HR. This is especially true if the skier suffers from asthma. The difficulties of distressed breathing from the combination of exercise in-

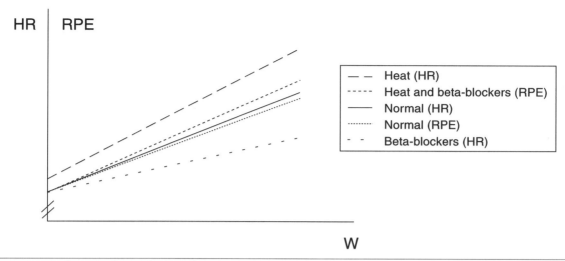

**Figure 10.1** A schematic figure showing the increase in HR and RPE with power (W) during different conditions (normal, heat, and beta blockers). For exercise in normal conditions there is a close relationship between HR and RPE both in slope and level. This is changed dramatically during the two abnormal conditions (heat and beta-blocker drugs) because HR increases or decreases, while RPE increases only slightly and still reflects mainly the actual exercise intensity.

tensity and cold may be very severe and cause an asthma attack.

Other important factors, such as altitude, noise, pollutants, and so on, seem to have a general effect on all people but also a differential effect (i.e., a greater effect on some people than others) depending on individual physiological or psychological differences. Music during exercise, such as during aerobic work, seems to change the HR-RPE relationship because changes in arousal or focus of attention decrease RPE.

An effect like that of music may be caused by a positive social environment. RPE depends not only on simple physiological signals, but also on emotional and motivational components. People exercising together in a comfortable environment may strain themselves harder without being aware of it. A typical case is that of the amateur downhill skier, who after two or three days of intense skiing (and improper eating and drinking) feels fatigued and stiff and suffers from lowered glycogen levels and reduced muscular strength. This person should stop skiing but does not listen to the body's signals because of the stimulating effect of friends and the nice environment. That extra run may be not only the last of the day, but also the last of the year.

If the day is hot and humid, a hard game of singles tennis against a slightly better opponent by a highly motivated underdog presents an increased risk of dangerous strain in the bodies of both athletes. This increased strain is important to perceive and, with luck, control. Appropriate perception of the components of the perceptual milieu will optimize competitive outcomes or the benefits of a rehabilitation program.

# Nutrition and Drugs

The influence of variations in food and liquid intake in terms of total calories and nutrient additives is not known as well as it should be. Moreover, the use of stimulants and sedative drugs and their effects on an individual's perception of effort needs further investigation. For example, it appears that moderate consumption of alcohol does not have a major impact on one's perception of effort during heavy exercise. In a study by Borg, Domserius, and Kaiser (1990) 10 men exercised on a bicycle ergometer with alcohol (1 g/kg body mass) and without alcohol (placebo). RPE did not differ, but HR significantly increased somewhat during exercise at the lowest power levels (50 W and 100 W).

The use of beta-blockers does not appear to greatly affect perceived exertion during exercise even though HR is reduced (figure 10.1). The effect depends, of course, on what kind, dosage, and combination of the medicine is taken. A study by Borg and colleagues (1972) found a significant effect of amphetamine and amobarbital on intermittent performance on the bicycle ergometer and the regression of the work (fatigue) curve. Blomstrand et al. (1997) found in a group of seven endurance-trained cyclists a decrease in perceived exertion (RPE) and mental fatigue (according to CR10 ratings) during cycling as an effect of ingestion of a special sports drink. This confirms many observations of a decreased RPE after a suitable drink during a marathon or a Vasa ski race.

While there is a need for more scientific investigations in this field, it is obvious that the psychophysiological relationships depend a great deal on factors such as those described in the preceding paragraphs. A common but mistaken belief is that the high correlations between RPE and HR found in so many studies depend mainly on the notion that people count their HR before giving their rating. That this is definitely wrong is evident, among other proofs, from the changes in the relationship between HR and RPE seen in figure 10.1.

# Physiological Factors

The variance observed in perceptual responses cannot be explained by one or even a few simple physiological factors. Among the factors most commonly used to explain this variance are HR, $\dot{V}O_2$, blood lactate, muscle lactate, blood pressure, ventilation and respiration rate, catecholamines, lactic acid, blood sugar, tissue temperature, and EMG. Many of the physiological correlates are unconscious reactions, but some are consciously perceived, such as HR, sweating, and respiration rate. Since ratings of perceived exertion for each individual give a direct, personally calibrated intensity level, it is not the absolute physiological measures, such as $\dot{V}O_2$, that are of major importance. Relative measures corresponding to each individual's maximum are better correlated to perceived exertion and can be used to predict the person's "absolute" perceptual intensity. It is interesting that relative HR (HR reserve) correlates better with RPE than do raw HR values (see Borg 1977).

## Effects of Sex

There has been some speculation about possible sex-related differences in RPE. It has commonly been found that, for the same physical exercise, women rate exertion significantly higher than men. Borg and Linderholm (1967, 1970) found,

however, that for work on the bicycle ergometer this common difference disappeared when relative measurements were compared and the exercise intensity was corrected according to working capacity. A similar result was obtained by Eston and Williams (1988), who found that exercise intensities corresponding to RPE 9, 13, and 17 did not differ between men and women.

## Effects of Age

Age is another important factor that may cause great differences in RPE responses. However, as in the case of sex, the main reason for these differences (at least for ordinary kinds of ergometer exercise) seems to be differences in working capacity. An exception to this rule has been found for children. This exception probably depends to a minor degree on somatic factors and to a major degree on cognitive factors and rating behavior. The extensive studies in Israel reported by Bar-Or (1977) found deviations from the normal age-related changes depending on increases in working capacity in children under 10 years old. Miyashita, Onodera, and Tabata (1986) found that Japanese children under 9 years old had difficulties using the RPE scale. Mahon and Marsh (1992) found large interindividual variability in RPE responses at the ventilatory threshold for 10-year-old American children. More studies about the use of RPE in children must be performed in order to understand the effects of rating behavior, instruction and training, personality, and motivation in different age groups and thus to know when and how to use the scale.

## Effects Due to Cognitive Abilities

When using the RPE scale in a simple ergometer test, 5% to 15% of the subjects in a normal population may have difficulties understanding the instructions and using the scale correctly. There are, however, few experiments in which related cognitive problems concerning rating behavior have been studied in terms of perceived exertion. More studies have been done focusing on other modalities and using psychophysical methods such as magnitude estimation (ME). These studies show that people differ not only in the way they understand instructions, but also in the way they use numbers. In ME the task is to try and represent relationships between intensities using numbers; some subjects prefer to use high numbers and others to use low numbers. When people use numbers in ME, they use them as personal conceptions and not as absolute mathematical concepts. This problem is partly a function of general psychological factors, but also of people's different attitudes toward and training in mathematics. Studies by Jones and Marcus (1961) and by Ekman et al. (1968) support the idea that perceptual judgments depend on a genuine, sensory, perceptual factor (based largely on physiological reactions) and on general human response behavior and individual response bias (rating behavior). Other studies have also shown contextual and methodological factors to have a significant influence on judgments (see Warren 1981 and Falmagne 1985).

The effect of cognitive factors such as intelligence (as measured by ordinary aptitude tests) has been studied by Borg and Borg (1992) in psychophysical studies of size perception using ME. The results showed that people who scored higher on aptitude tests, were well-educated, and had a good knowledge of mathematics obtained higher exponents and showed lower variability. Even if there are no extensive studies of this kind concerning perceived exertion, there is no reason to believe that similar results would not be obtained since many given ratings depend on the individual's rating behavior. The construction of the RPE scale and the CR10 scale (with numbers and verbal expressions well anchored according to the instruction and a fundamental inner frame of reference) should, however, minimize the effect of intelligence or rating behavior in studies of perceived exertion.

Cognitive, linguistic factors are of great importance for perception and correct identification of objects and events. The final stage in most perceptual tasks is naming an object. Verbal descriptions also seem to affect the actual nature of the perception, so that those features represented by linguistic terms stand out in greater perceptual articulation. The relationship between perception and language has been studied thoroughly in visual perception ever since the early stages of experimental psychology (see Vernon 1962). The influence of naming is also strong in the reproduction of visually perceived forms from memory.

Many findings in visual perception also seem to be valid in other fields of perception, such as perceived effort and exertion. There is, however, no strong experimental evidence from the area of perceived exertion about how the use of language and the ability to name a subjective, somatic symptom facilitates perception and identification. It is probably true that, in this case as well, we tend to perceive most readily that which we can name most easily. This should therefore be true not only for qualitative aspects of exertion or pain, but also for quantitative aspects.

To discriminate between different levels of intensities, we need good verbal anchors. Rating scales such as the Borg RPE scale or the Borg CR10 scale give good reference points for identification. This feature of the scales should also help scale

## A Good Name Helps You Identify Things

A problem that fascinated me in high school was the importance of naming things. I read in a popular psychology book that in the final stage of perceiving something it is important to be able to associate a name with the object or event. In this way the object is not only better remembered, but also easier to perceive and identify.

I had a biology teacher who was a specialist in birds; he liked to take us out in the woods on excursions to see birds and flowers. He could name many different kinds, and it was indeed fascinating to see how many he could detect and identify when most of us didn't see anything or only a few. He could also point out the main differences among the types of snow like an Eskimo, who can discriminate among 100 different kinds.

When I started with my studies of perceived exertion, I thus thought it important to be able to identify and name different kinds of exertion, such as "pedal resistance," "muscle fatigue," "muscle pain," "joint pain" (of many kinds), "normal breathlessness," and "abnormal breathlessness." I also thought that it would be valuable to train and reinforce the use of the right adjectives and adverbs for different levels of intensity.

users produce and monitor performances in accordance with the requirements or goals of a certain situation. This is especially important for submaximal performances, where too much or too little effort spoils everything. As examples, consider the optimal amount of effort required for a golf putt, a kick in soccer, or a jump shot in basketball.

# Psychological Factors

Perceived exertion and its variation within and among individuals depends not only on the intensity of the exercise or other physical factors in the environment or the context, but also on psychological factors. Most of the variance in perceived exertion (more in the form of the inner sensory perception than the given RPE responses) can be "explained" by physical and physiological factors such as those described in the preceding sections. (I place the word "explained" within quotation marks here to denote that it is not a causal, but rather a correlational, explanation.) But still a rather large part of the variance depends on other factors, especially psychological factors, such as the subject's motivation, emotional state, and personality.

## Motivation

The motivation of the subject is an important psychological factor. Well-motivated people, such as athletes, commonly tend to underestimate their perceived exertion in relation to ordinary people. They are not only proud of being fit and performing at the extreme of their ability, they are also used to such performances and have a more positive attitude toward them. The habit of straining yourself to the utmost changes your frame of reference and gives mental representations and anchors that are higher than usual. In a test on very young, competitive Swedish tennis players (Borg, unpublished data), most of the subjects underestimated perceived exertion in relation to their working capacity. When this study was performed at the end of the 1970s, these athletes knew they were among the best in the world in their age group, and they did not want to admit that they were as tired as they actually were. This may, however, be a rather bad tactic or defense mechanism, since it may mean that they are more likely to overstrain themselves.

The opposite tendency—to overestimate actual exertion—is also rather common. A low degree of motivation for exercise in general or for a particular kind of exercise usually causes subjects to overestimate the intensity. People with a negative attitude toward exercise and who are not used to straining themselves may also be afraid of somatic damage. Low motivation goes hand in hand with negative feelings and task aversion, which affect RPE responses.

Physical exercise and perceived exertion provide an extraordinary opportunity for estimating a subject's degree of achievement motivation by looking at the relationship between physical resources and performances. If physical endowments are correctly measured and used as an independent variable and a predictor of performance, and an actual maximal performance is used as the dependent variable, a regression function can be obtained for the normal cases. Deviations above and below the normal function can be interpreted as differences in individual motivation. During very extreme performances, however, motivated individuals may show decreased performance, especially in activities highly dependent on good technique and psychomotor coordination. An extreme subjective effort to perform well, which results in a similarly extreme perceived exertion for the performance, may thus be detrimental to performance in some sports.

## Emotional State

Stable emotional factors or temporary moods, such as depression, anxiety, anger, or delight, can also influence ratings of perceived exertion. This is especially obvious in some clinical cases, such as in patients with cardiopulmonary diseases who are afraid of overstraining themselves. In rehabilitation of cardiac patients after an infarction or bypass surgery, it is important to slowly get the individual accustomed to an appropriate level of exercise intensity. In this way, patients do not have to worry about the moderate exercise to be performed and do not feel that they are being forced to exercise at a dangerous level. For people in a state of depression, most activities may be difficult to perform and feel heavy (Borg 1962a). Healthy, active people who enjoy exercising, on the other hand, may not feel the real exertion, but instead underestimate its magnitude.

In all clinical cases involving patients with somatic or psychological disorders, it is especially important to fully and correctly inform patients of the significance of appropriate levels of exercise. If they are not convinced that the exercise is vital for their health and well-being, they may be very suspicious of physical activities. Thus, during an exercise test they may feel that they are being forced to exercise too much and at an intensity level that they may judge to be dangerous. They may then give a high RPE value to escape a risky situation.

In some hospitals and rehabilitation centers, test leaders have noticed that some patients seem to decide before the test that they will give a high rating soon after the beginning of the test, even if the exertion is not especially high. If a test leader has good reasons to believe that this might be the case, he or she must work harder to inform, convince, and motivate the person. It is necessary at this point to get the person more involved in the testing procedure. It may be a good idea to avoid a rigid time-workload schedule in which the test leader sets the resistance and the patient is passively tested, and instead to let the patient set the resistance and monitor changes slowly. Thus the patient is not forced to respond to a given load but can set a load that corresponds to a preferred intensity and a given RPE level. In this way, the patient may develop a sense of control over the situation and gradually become less afraid and more motivated.

The best and most secure way of monitoring exercise intensity is to use as much information as possible from all three of the effort continua: physiological responses such as those obtained by ECG and so on, perceptual responses such as perceived exertion and perceived speed, and performance responses such as workload, velocity, and time. One kind of information channel taken alone may give somewhat misleading results. You cannot detect all somatic weaknesses using ECG or RPE; silent symptoms might be lying in wait. To collect and integrate all the information of possible importance would, however, be very circumstantial and impractical. It might also be stressful for the person being tested and might not involve the good subjectivity that can be obtained using the RPE scale.

If there are no observable signs or symptoms of danger, we can be reasonably sure that we do not need to worry about exercising at a prescribed intensity level. But we can never be completely certain about the presence of unobservable pathological disorders. Avoiding exercise because of anxiety about silent symptoms is, however, a bad strategy in the long run. To keep fit, we do not

need to exercise at high intensity levels but can, to a large degree, trade intensity for total amount (frequency and duration) of exercise.

## Personality Factors

Several studies have observed that personality factors influence perceived exertion (see Rejeski 1985). Morgan (1973) showed that people who received a kind of hypnotic suggestion of heavy work rated the exertion to be higher than normal. Morgan was also one of the first to study attentional factors and association and dissociation (Morgan and Pollock 1977). In the model by Kinsman and Weiser (1975) and Pandolf (1975), motivation and task aversion play an important role. Dishman and co-workers (1991) did not find support for the hypothesis that type A behavior predicts perceived exertion during exercise. (Type A refers to a person with excessive drive, time urgency, ambition, impatience, aggressiveness, hostility, and competitiveness, as measured by the Bortner scale.) The study was well designed, but the kind and intensity of exercise was not very stressing. In contrast, Hassmén, Ståhl, and Borg (1993) found that men with this type A trait tended to perform about the same as others but to underestimate perceived exertion when performing a harder and more challenging run test on an outdoor track (see figure 10.2).

There are few hard facts about the relationship between personality and RPE responses. In my laboratory at Stockholm University we are now conducting further experiments on personality and perceived exertion. The study on type A personality and perceived exertion has been enlarged

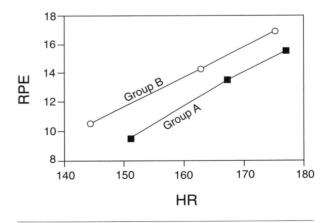

**Figure 10.2** The relationship between RPE and HR in type A individuals (group A) and non–type A individuals (group B) according to Hassmén, Ståhl, and Borg 1993.

with experiments including many personality factors, such as trait and state anxiety, according to Spielberger (1975) and Eysenck's three PEN factors (psychoticism, extroversion, and neuroticism; Eysenck 1994). It should also be interesting to study the effect on RPE of the "big five" factors, traditionally labeled (I) surgency (or extroversion), (II) agreeableness, (III) conscientiousness (or dependability), (IV) emotional stability (vs. neuroticism), and (V) culture (or intellect) (see Halverson, Kohnstamm, and Martin 1994; Costa and Widiger 1994). Preliminary results from our lab show a possible sex-related effect, indicating that extroverted and aggressive women—contrary to type A men—perform better than their less extreme female counterparts, but at a higher "perceptual" cost (higher and probably more valid RPE). The issue of whether women are more or less sensitive raters of perceived exertion than men, however, is still an open question.

# Weighing All the Factors

Many important problems in the field of perceived exertion are illustrated and discussed in this chapter. Quite a few studies have been carried out, but several of them are of substandard quality. Many better studies have to be performed to make valid generalizations possible. One reason for the rather weak development in this area is the many difficulties involved in carrying out good studies. The field is very difficult to explore because so many different physiological and psychological factors interact. Moreover, these factors are at work during vastly different actions and situations, with performances varying from explosive strength exertion to long-term endurance exertion to intermittent or continuous exercise with differences in performance patterns over time, all taking place in different physical and social contexts. Designing good experiments also is difficult because of the indistinctness of personality theories and methods. Ongoing development of the field of psychology of personality, however, will hopefully result in more and higher-quality studies in the RPE field. I know personally that some of my colleagues and students are occupied with studies about RPE and such personality factors as introversion and extroversion, trait and state anxiety, type A behavior, and possible differences between men and women. Unfortunately, there are few studies that

have dealt with sex-related issues and psychophysiological comparisons.

It is difficult to summarize which factors are the most important and should be given the most weight when attempting to "explain" the variation of RPE responses. Physiological factors related to measurements of working capacity are, however, very important and may account for most of the variance. In a population including many people with cardiopulmonary or musculoskeletal disorders, pathological symptoms are especially important. Among the psychological factors, individual rating behavior (which depends mostly on cognitive abilities and personality factors) may be most important. Motivational and emotional factors influence the balance and accuracy of estimations and are certainly quite important. For example, extreme judgments may result from repression or denial of the perception or from the opposite, exaggeration and symptom magnification.

If we do not use the Borg RPE scale as a differential test to study perceived exertion from a differential point of view, but use it rather as a way of obtaining a general S-R function that is valid for most individuals, we can conclude that HR is the best single predictor for the variation of RPE over exercise intensities (and vice versa). When using ratio scaling methods and the Borg CR10 scale, on the other hand, the best and simplest prediction of perceptual responses is obtained by integrating measurements of both HR and blood lactate.

It will be a great challenge for researchers in this field to further explore the importance of psychological factors for RPE. I don't know of any other field in psychology or psychophysiology in which so many relevant physiological factors can be used for predictions of a perceptual response. If we define the physiological variables as independent variables and use them to predict the RPE responses as a dependent variable, we should obtain high correlations. Depending on the kind of activity, situation, and so on, however, we will get deviations from the prediction that should depend greatly on individual psychological factors. By using such a research strategy and as many relevant and reliable predictors as possible, for example, by using multiple regression analysis, we can create unusually good opportunities for obtaining a clearer and more detailed picture of the meaning of RPE and its physiological and psychological components.

# Chapter 11

## Applying the Scales to Training and Rehabilitation

When a person performs any kind of exercise or rehabilitation program, it is important that he or she pay attention to several perceptual cues, including overall perceived exertion, breathlessness, chest pain, fatigue in the working muscles, or aches in the joints. Many other perceptual cues relate to the physical environment and to inner emotional and motivational factors.

When we exercise, it is important to feel good and enjoy the activity. We can all stand physical or mental stress if it is combined with a feeling of well-being and not accompanied by severe negative feelings of anxiety or fear. A physical activity that is enjoyable is also healthier and makes us more motivated to continue exercising.

Since the 1960s there has been a great increase in scientific knowledge based on the research in sport sciences. This knowledge is of great help not only for top athletes and their training (see chapter 13) but also for common people who are training to improve health and fitness, lose weight, or rehabilitate after an injury or illness.

In planning an individual's training or rehabilitation program, it is important to integrate information about the individual from the three effort continua (defined in chapter 1): the perceptual, the physiological, and the performance-based. Meeting this need is also important to improve an individual's motivation to take part and be active throughout his or her lifetime. Too many people start to exercise but after a short time drop out. By integrating perceptual cues in a feedback system, effective, lifelong training models may become less rigid and more individualized and motivate people to continue exercising.

There are many good books and articles as well as coaches, doctors, physiologists, and therapists that can give good advice about how to exercise. Anyone interested in starting to exercise should acquire some basic information concerning mode, duration, frequency, and intensity of exercise from a reputable source such as the American College of Sports Medicine (ACSM). Sources such as these give ideas and guidelines about the type of exercise and how much and how often an individual should exercise based on his or her fitness or health goals. The intensity of exercise is also important but is more difficult to determine since it depends on an individual's health status, the aim and mode of the exercise, and the total physical and cultural context. Due to these various factors that influence exercise intensity, perceptual factors, such as perceived exertion, are especially important to consider (Pollock, Jackson, and Foster 1986; Capodaglio and Capodaglio 1995; Noble and Robertson 1996).

## Mode of Exercise

Many general fitness books focus exclusively on specialty activities, such as running, bicycling, weight training, or aerobic workouts. These activities are fine, but don't underestimate the importance of ordinary daily activities such as walking, shopping, gardening, bicycling, cleaning the house, and so on. There are great cultural differences in these basic physical activities. In

---

## A Smörgåsbord *of Exercises*

Personally, I think the best exercise is like a *smörgåsbord*—a table with many dishes from vegetables to meat, from cold to hot, and so on—from which you eat *lagom* (just the right amount). Your *smörgåsbord* of exercise should consist of many things: an active daily life at home, at work, and in your garden; playing with your children; and also some special training activities, such as running, swimming, or weight training. You will enjoy this *smörgåsbord* if you do not eat it all but select the right items; take it easy; do not eat too fast, too much, or too little; and stop before you are too full.

---

the Nordic countries it is common in the summer to pick berries or mushrooms in the woods, take part in orienteering, or just take a bicycle ride to buy a newspaper. In winter it is common to go downhill skiing in the mountains, cross-country skiing in the nearby woods, or skating on one of the hundreds of thousands of lakes and fjords. It is thus popular to *gå på tur* (take a nice walk in the woods) as the Norwegians say, not really with the intent to train but just to be active and do something nice with the family. Most of these activities take several hours but are still perceived as enjoyable. Even if the intensity isn't high, the total duration of activity is long and can improve one's fitness and ability to control weight.

To add variety to a physical fitness program, add some favorite aerobic activities to your daily or weekend activities. The simplest things are often the best, such as running, swimming, and organized workouts. To adhere to an activity over a long period of time, it is important to select something that you enjoy. Games such as tennis, basketball, volleyball, football, soccer, and so on are good sports that can be enjoyed with others.

Perceptual cues are important in all of these activities. Differences in perceived exertion among modes of exercise can affect a person's degree of motivation. For example, if an individual chooses to start running, he or she must know that it may take some time before it will be enjoyable. At first the person may find that the activity is boring, is too hard, has too many disturbing perceptual cues from the environment, or causes unpleasant bodily sensations of strain and discomfort. After adjusting to running, however, the individual may forget about many of these cues and difficulties and may enjoy it. Performing an aerobic workout with pleasant music in an enjoyable social context also may diminish perceived exertion and facilitate performance.

# Frequency and Duration of Exercise

Common advice regarding exercise frequency is to engage in exercise above your training threshold three to four times a week. If you usually devote yourself to activities during the weekend, such as walking, cycling, hiking, golf, or tennis, do more specific aerobic training (running or aerobic workouts) on Tuesdays and Thursdays. If your weekend activities don't give you much aerobic training, exercise three days during the week and add some activity during the weekend.

The duration of an activity may be more problematic for the novice exerciser. Common advice when an individual starts a program after a long period of inactivity is to not exercise more than 10 to 15 min per session. This general advice may be misleading because it underestimates the importance of learning the activity in question and its context. Depending on the individual and the mode of exercise—whether it is continuous or intermittent, is performed alone or in a group, has the character of a game or not, and so on—the duration may vary greatly.

In choosing the right frequency and duration, a person's perception of exertion and difficulty can help him or her regulate the activity according to what feels just right. If the individual's main goal in being physically active is to lose weight rather than to improve aerobic capacity, training intensity can be traded for amount (duration and frequency) of exercise.

# Intensity of Exercise

The most difficult thing to give good advice about is the exercise intensity level; the "right" intensity is not constant, but depends on a combination of mode, frequency, and duration of exercise as well as environmental conditions, such as whether it is hot or humid; the age, sex, and health and fitness of the individual; and the goal of the exercise (Blair and Connolly 1994). Recommended exercise intensity varies, depending on the target group: top athletes, ordinary people used to exercise, novices, overweight people, people with cardiovascular or pulmonary diseases or musculoskeletal disorders, or people with psychological or psychiatric problems.

However, if we do not start from a general model, it is difficult to give any advice at all; thus a general model to suit a large group of healthy people is necessary. From this model, deviations can be proposed to suit individuals. The model should not be too rigid but should encourage the individual to follow a schematic procedure. Include the perception of exertion and other psychological cues to make it easier to adapt the training to special, temporary factors, such as feelings of discomfort because of a slight infection, a knee that hurts, and so on.

Most models for good aerobic training start from "absolute" physiological factors and functioning. One model—for which it is not necessary to measure $\dot{V}O_2$, blood lactate, or other parameters—utilizes HR, since HR grows linearly with $\dot{V}O_2$ and power for most heavy exercises, such as running and cycling. For an exercise to have a good aerobic fitness effect, the exercise intensity is recommended to be between 50% to 85% of maximal aerobic capacity (ACSM 1991). The HR at these levels is about 65% to 90% of the maximal HR of an individual (see chapter 5) or 50% to 85% of the relative HR (see chapter 8). For each individual a special target HR level can be chosen that fits the mode of exercise in question. For people with physical disorders a lower intensity is recommended. When they have recovered enough to take part in a supervised exercise program, the lower value may be around 40% of maximum. Recent research by Blair and Connolly (1994) showed that this level may also have a training effect for healthy people.

A drawback with using only HR as the variable for the target intensity is that the maximal HR and resting HR for an individual are sometimes difficult to determine. This makes the target HR rather uncertain. Another problem is that, depending on the mode of exercise, there may be a time lag in HR response to exercise, such as during short-term, intermittent exercise. A special drawback is that people who are exercising using feedback signals from HR tend to become somewhat compulsive HR counters and cannot really enjoy the exercise because they are always checking their HR, afraid of deviations from the target.

People who have learned to use the RPE scale and tested themselves in a laboratory test or field test can effectively use the scale to select an appropriate training intensity. The linearity between HR and RPE facilitates the choice of a good target RPE level without relying on knowing one's HR at all times. From many exercise tests we know the relationship between RPE and HR and other physiological variables, such as $\dot{V}O_2$ and blood lactate. We therefore do not have to worry much about selecting a good RPE value. From several studies we also know how perceived exertion changes with age in relation to HR (see figure 11.1). It is always good to try to combine a target HR model with a target RPE model to utilize the advantages and avoid the drawbacks of both models.

For ordinary people to train successfully according to the Borg RPE scale, a training model has to be simple. Models that are too complicated can be confusing or make people postpone exercise until they have time to read all the instructions! Rather, people should learn how the scale functions, check how it fits with their knowledge about training and their own HR, then follow their feelings. It is important for an individual to know that he or she is in good health and does not have any heart or other medical problems. If the exercise doesn't feel too hard and is enjoyable, then it is okay. A beginner should start by taking it very easy and keeping the intensity low (between 9 and 13 on the scale).

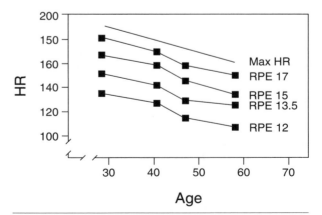

**Figure 11.1** The decrease with age in maximal HR and HR for different RPE levels (after Borg and Linderholm 1967).

As he or she becomes more accustomed to the exercise and feels comfortable, he or she may increase the intensity to between 11 and 15. If running outdoors on a hilly trail, it may also be natural to vary the intensity and run a bit harder uphill and take it easier downhill (this is also better for the joints). Athletes who want to train more intensely must not be afraid of training up to, or close to, their maximum (see chapter 13).

It is important, of course, that people with physical disorders do not exercise too hard. Depending on the disease and the stage in rehabilitation, choose duration and intensity level carefully. This is also important for ordinarily healthy people with slight infections or who just don't feel well. If your doctor gives you advice to exercise carefully at a low intensity, pay special attention to your body's symptoms. Slow down as soon as you feel too much strain, and cut down the exercise duration. Unfortunately, there are always some people who overdo it and train too hard, even if they have an infection or don't feel well. Their health and training might subsequently suffer. The RPE scale is a good tool to help an individual regulate exercise intensity and not overdo it.

# Short-Term Exercise and Muscular Training

Studies of perceived effort and exertion have not been as common in short-term exercise (of duration up to a minute) as in long-term (many minutes) aerobic exercise. This is unfortunate, since many fundamental experiments could be performed to elucidate theoretical psychophysiological relationships. Many applications in training and ergonomics, such as manual materials handling (see chapter 12), also concern short-term activities. The perception during activities that last from parts of a second up to a minute is accurate and does not have the time lag that many physiological responses (e.g., HR or blood lactate) have. Like EMG measurements, the perception of exertion (or subjective force) is an immediate response. An advantage of perception is that it integrates many cues and is easy to obtain. For well-instructed and competent individuals it also has a built-in individual calibration since it reflects the exercise intensity relative to their individual capacity.

The first studies on perceived exertion dealt with short-term exercise on the bicycle ergometer (Borg and Dahlström 1959, 1960; see chapter 4). The problem was to try to find out whether there are any consistent relationships between perceived exertion and relevant physical variables. We knew that for this kind of continuous exercise with simple movement patterns, the elementary physical laws could be applied, namely, power is work (energy) divided by time and work is force multiplied by time and pedaling speed. What relationship exists between the physical parameters and the perceived magnitude was unknown, however, and is still mostly unknown. For pedaling speed we know that there may be a special effect that depends on changes in mechanical efficiency. People seem to prefer and be most comfortable with a speed around 50 to 60 rpm. It therefore presumably should be true that this is the most economical rate with the lowest costs physiologically and mentally. However, racing cyclists usually prefer a somewhat higher pedaling speed.

Better knowledge of these functions should be helpful in several situations, for example, in muscular training and dose-response moderation. A person who comes to a gym for fitness training using modern exercise machines for different muscle groups may find it difficult to choose just the right weight for a certain number of sets and repetitions within each set. The inexperienced person needs a simple method to help select the right starting weight that after a certain number of repetitions will give the desired and suitable end result for the set in question. My proposition to solve this problem is to use the following five-step procedure:

1. Get acquainted with the rating scale, the Borg RPE scale or the Borg CR10 scale.

2. Choose a desired endpoint or goal on the scale that you should reach after the recommended number of repetitions.

3. Use a chart that gives the suitable rating value that you should perceive for the first weight in order to reach the target rating at the end of the set. Figure 11.2 is an example of such a chart for 12 reps using the CR10 scale. For instance, if your target rating at the end of the set is 6 ("hard" to "very hard"), you should rate the first rep 3 ("moderate") according to the chart.

4. Determine the weight to start with by testing a few weights, starting with one that

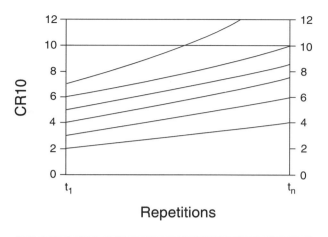

**Figure 11.2** How to select an initial and target intensity in weight training using perception of force and fatigue ($t_1$ = the first repetition and $t_n$ = the last of a number of reps, in this case 12).

seems about right, but slightly lighter. Lift it for two reps and give a rating. If you rate the exertion lower than indicated by the chart, increase the weight and do another two reps, continuing this process until you have found the right starting level. If you rate the first two reps too high, proceed as described except with decreasing weight.

5. Do the total numbers of reps using the determined starting weight. If you reach your target rating before achieving the desired number of reps, or if you do not achieve your target rating, change the starting weight as appropriate.

There is currently no well-established chart that can be used in the process. Probably different charts are needed for different exercises, situations, and groups of subjects. Figure 11.2 provides a preliminary chart of 12 repetitions as an example of what such a chart might look like for weight lifting. Depending on the muscle groups to be trained, the total exercise time, the number of sets, and so on, you must further modify your weights.

# Long-Term Exercise Regulation

When a person has been training for a long time and has adapted to the mode, duration, fre-

quency, intensity, and all other aspects of exercise, it may be natural to slightly change the training model. Maybe the person will try some other activities or increase the intensity and the RPE target. Depending on the person's exercising goals, it may be time to take a good exercise test to check changes in aerobic fitness, muscular strength, or flexibility. Periodically checking fitness gives important information about how to regulate training. Seeing the improvements on a personal chart is also recognized as very motivating. You can test your aerobic fitness by using the simple run test presented in chapter 8.

In some cases regulation may mean not an increase in intensity, but a decrease because of strain in the working muscles and joints, overtraining, or feelings of discomfort. It is seldom wise to make abrupt changes or to interrupt an exercise program if not necessary because of injuries. A gradual, long-term regulation is often advantageous.

# Rehabilitation

For patients who have been severely sick and still have to be careful about their physical activities, it is important to use RPE with sound judgment. These patients must follow the prescriptions from their doctors and use all their doctor's information and advice, not only perceptual cues.

When a cardiopulmonary or musculoskeletal patient recovers enough to start exercising more intensely, any of the training models described in preceding sections are applicable. In a rehabilitation program—for instance, after a myocardial infarction—the patient should learn to exercise and experience appropriate intensity levels according to HR and RPE. When the patient is allowed to return home from the hospital, he or she can then rely on HR and RPE to monitor exercise and exertion. Exercise should be started with an RPE no higher than 9 to 11, then after a while progress up to about 13. Remember, when exercise is "hard" (15), it is too hard.

For good quality of life a person should not have to rely on apparatuses and physiological recordings; rather a person should be able to follow his or her own perception of somatic symptoms. It should be possible to live a normal life, work in the household, make love, work in the garden, and so on at an appropriate intensity level. At the same time it is important that a person with a chronic disorder attend to special signs and symptoms that should signal him or her to slow down or stop and that he or she follow prescriptions and the individualized rehabilitation program. After a long recovery period some people with chronic disorders may exercise harder than others and thus may work at an intensity level usual for most healthy people.

However, it is better for a person not to strain him- or herself too much, but to take it easy and to exchange intensity for amount of exercise, for example, to take a good brisk walk for an hour instead of running fast for 20 minutes. All training models, including the RPE model, can present some danger. The exercising person may not perceive silent signs of a heart disorder. However, in the long run, exercising sensibly is a better alternative than avoiding exercise altogether.

# Chapter 12

# Ergonomics and Epidemiology

Ergonomics and epidemiology are two scientific fields that have a strong focus on applications using a combination of physiological and psychological (and technological) methods. The fields have much in common and are therefore dealt with in one chapter. Both fields study the effect of daily activities and the environment (in a broad sense, referring to global and local situations, the milieu and living conditions, and the work tasks and tools in daily work and leisure-time activities) on measures of performance, working capacity, health, and disease. They also study how improvements in situational factors can be carried out to produce benefits for the individual or his or her daily activities and work tasks. The main interest in both these fields is measuring intensity of exposure and degrees of difficulty. Often similar questionnaire methods are used concerning the interaction between the individual and his or her situation. Questionnaires often include ratings of subjective somatic symptoms and relevant feelings.

Epidemiology is interested in the effect of the environment on people's health, while in ergonomics the interest is not focused on people per se, but on situations: "consumer friendliness" and possibilities to make technical improvements. In both fields subjective evaluations of activity-related exposures are fundamental. However, ergonomics is task- and situation-oriented, and epidemiology is people- or individual-oriented.

Human beings are built for physical and mental work, though modern society's demands are typically more mental than physical. We are overwhelmed by information and sensory stimuli and must carefully select those most relevant for performance, often in a stressing situation, such as driving in heavy traffic. We seem to be paying for these environmental and social changes not only with declining physical fitness, but also with an increase in circulatory diseases and psychological stress symptoms.

In spite of the diminishing demands on physical achievements in performing daily work tasks, one of the most important causes of poor health and work-related disease and complaints is still physical load (according to the Swedish Labor Union). That this is the case in modern industry may be astonishing and alarming, since it was thought that modern machines would protect humans from damage caused by physical load and manual materials handling. However, even though physically stressing work tasks are not as heavy as they once were, they are now highly repetitive and performed in static or extreme positions. Even if they are of a low intensity, they may therefore still cause severe work-related injuries.

## Ergonomics

In ergonomics (human factors engineering) using psychophysical methods for subjectively evaluating work tasks and determining acceptable loads has become rather common. Daily activities at the work site (lifting, carrying, and tasks done in various positions) and at home (housework, gardening, etc.) are studied not only with physiological methods but also with perceptual estimation and production methods to better understand and solve ergonomic problems. The psychophysical methods are of special interest in field studies of short-term work tasks for which valid physiological measurements are difficult to obtain.

The perceived exertion, difficulty, and fatigue that a person experiences in a certain work situation is, as a rule, an important sign of a real or objective load. Measurement of the physical load is not sufficient since it does not take into consideration the particular difficulty of the performance or the capacity of the individual. It is often difficult from technical and biomechanical analyses to understand the seriousness of a difficulty that a person experiences. Physiological determinations give important information, but they may be insufficient due to technical problems in obtaining relevant but simple measurements for short-term activities or activities involving special movement patterns.

Perceptual estimations give important information because the severity of a task's difficulty depends on the individual doing the work. The worker may have an incipient disease or other disorder or may be especially sensitive to the work task or situation in question. If, however, several people at the work site perceive the same stress and there are no signs of physical illness or disease among these individuals, the work situation has to be searched for the reason. Feeling well and being able to perform a work task without complaints and symptoms of illness are important not only for the individual, but also, in the long run, for the industry or company in question to avoid absentees, keep production steady, and create a good social climate.

To understand the strain a person is exposed to during work it is important to listen to the worker's own experiences of difficulties and not simply to observe the worker, work task, environment, performances, and physiological responses. It is important to pay attention to the costs—both in the form of mental and physiological responses—behind the performances. Extensive methodological studies using subjective evaluations in manual materials handling (MMH) and acceptable loads have been performed by Ayoub (1986), Ashfour et al. (1983), and Gamberale (1990). Studies by Fleishman et al. (1986) and Capodaglio, Capodaglio, and Bazzini (1995) helped bridge the gap between psychophysical studies and physiological ones in the field of applied ergonomics.

A good method is essential for subjective evaluations. In several investigations we have found that both the Borg RPE scale and the Borg CR10 scale may function well for subjective estimations. If the work task's demand is mainly physical, the RPE scale has often been used. If the problem more concerns mental tasks or a combination of mental difficulty and physical strain, the CR10 scale may be more appropriate.

In a production method the worker may be asked to perform the task at a suitable pace with loads selected by the worker as acceptable or preferred. It is often possible to select tasks and intensity levels that have a natural relevance for the individual and the work task in question. The subjects should be well-experienced workers in order to obtain valid results and draw sound conclusions.

Interestingly, the International Organization for Standardization (ISO) in 1981 accepted the following principle with regard to work tasks and situations:

> The work environment shall be designed and maintained so that physical, chemical and biological conditions have no noxious effect on people but serve to ensure their health, as well as their capacity and readiness to work. Account shall be taken of objectively measurable phenomena and of subjective assessments. (International Organization for Standardization 1981)

Since the ISO accepted this principle, it is important also to agree on some standardized methods for "subjective assessments."

When a special product or work task is to be evaluated, selecting a relevant group of subjects for the study and defining the difficulties of the task and the variables for the evaluation are important (e.g., how easy it is to handle a product, how easy it is to avoid or to make errors, how fast and correctly the task can be performed, how well the task fits into the context, what complaints workers have, what kind of collaboration is needed, how long it takes to learn to use the tool or the product, etc.). The subjects in a special test situation should be well instructed about the problem and what they are supposed to do; they should get detailed information of the test method, including the scale to be used; and preferably they should be trained in using the scale with special test material.

Many field studies have been performed using the RPE scale or the CR10 scale. A study by Johansson and Ljunggren (1989) collected both

## Some Problems in Ergonomics

Dr. Peter Holzmann and I made an interesting use of subjective evaluations according to the CR10 scale. This application concerned the construction of some technical devices used for milking machines. People using these milking machines experienced some difficulty with the handles when putting the nozzle into the hole or taking it out (as when filling up a car with gas). We were asked to study different apparatuses and make a subjective evaluation of the difficulties.

Since physiological and performance measurements are difficult to use, and in some situations neither valid nor informative, we used our subjective evaluation technique. We analyzed the performances in detail and identified the different movements or movement patterns and the difficulties with them. Holding the handle well, fitting it securely into the hole, releasing it, taking it off, and cleaning it caused difficulties that depended on special handling problems, the heaviness of the apparatus, and other factors. About five different variables were identified, and all were used in the subjective evaluations. Subjects rated the difficulty of the task (in each variable) according to the CR10 scale. The profiles of ratings for the different apparatuses thus obtained gave good information about the main difficulties, which of the products was best, and what needed improvement.

HR and CR10 measures in a group of female cleaners performing their ordinary work. The results showed that the level of exertion was rather high and corresponded to about 35% of estimated $\dot{V}O_2$max. Back symptoms were found in most subjects, but there were also symptoms in the neck, shoulders, wrists, and hands, indicating the performances that were most critical.

In a similar field study of male tank truck drivers, Johansson and Borg (1993) evaluated different phases of the heavy work operations. The researchers identified many difficulties of interest for comparisons of both individuals and work tasks. With the help of the CR10 scale the difficulties of tanking (including pulling out the hose, pulling in the hose, connecting the hose, etc.) were studied. The heaviest work was pulling out the hose, which resulted in ratings ranging from 1 to 10, with a mean value of 3.2, and corresponding HRs varying from 110 to 169 bpm, with a mean value of 137 bpm. Other stressors for the truck drivers were noise, vibration, draft, heat, and the exhaust gases in traffic. The ratings of the work operations show potential health problems and the need for ergonomic improvements.

In one of the most recent studies of MMH, involving a group of wood cutters, Hagen (1994) used RPE with physiological measurements to evaluate technical improvements in certain tools and to compare different lifting techniques. In one part of the study the squat technique and the stoop technique for repetitive lifting were investigated in 10 male forest workers. One conclusion was that "relative RPE was more accurate than relative $VO_2$ for determining the relative aerobic intensity in repetitive lifting." It was also concluded that "the stoop technique is not superior to the squat technique in terms of central perceived exertion" (Hagen 1994).

In many ergonomic work studies it is not the worker him- or herself who judges the difficulty. Instead a foreman or a panel of experts following the worker at work makes this judgment. Some of these studies use psychophysical scaling methods. Ljunggren (1986) collected RPE values from observer ratings of MMH, and Holzmann (1982) videotaped several work operations, identified different dimensions of workload and strain, and quantified the intensities in each dimension using the CR10 scale when analyzing the videotapes.

It is important that ergonomic evaluations be used to improve the work, not to select workers. While in some cases it may be important to select people with certain qualities for specific jobs (e.g., firefighters who are strong or pilots with good stress tolerance), it is not only bad practice to select only certain people (e.g., men instead of women, younger persons instead of older) if the work task can be adapted to suit most people, it may also be illegal, as in the United States.

# Epidemiological Intensity Evaluations

A less-developed field for perceptual evaluations involving physical activity is in epidemiological investigations. In interviews and questionnaire studies of the health status of different populations, information pertaining to the kind and frequency of activities of populations is commonly assembled, but little information is obtained concerning the intensity of these activities. To illustrate the problems, I'll take examples from sports.

Exercises such as running, bicycling, and swimming are excellent activities for aerobic training, and their training response is recognized to be equivalent (figure 12.1). Tennis and badminton, on the other hand, are examples of sports that motivate many people physically, mentally, and socially, but that are not as aerobically demanding as bicycling. Many daily activities at home, in the garden, or at work are also physically demanding. A certain sport's or daily activity's potential for a high training

response (as determined, for example, by studying athletes' demands and responses) and its actual training effect for ordinary people must be distinguished since these activities often are done only for pleasure and not for physical training.

In a Swedish SIFO investigation (similar to a Gallup survey) a representative sample of men and women in the greater Stockholm area were asked to retrospectively rate the RPE of their usual leisure-time activities (Borg, Edgren, and Levin 1978; Borg 1986). Those who exercised regularly (10% to 20% of the sample) judged running to be the most aerobically demanding of the activities studied, with RPE values estimated at 15 ("hard"). Football (called soccer in the United States), badminton, and tennis were also among the activities rated at 14 (almost "hard"). Swimming and bicycling were rated lower, approximately 13. These results may be typical for Swedish men and women.

These findings suggest that the intensity of an activity should be judged not only in terms of its type and potential for training, but also according to general and individual differences in exer-

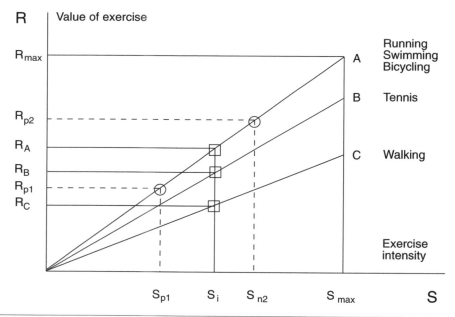

**Figure 12.1** How exercise value (R) varies with exercise intensity (S) for three different kinds of activities. The same exercise intensity ($S_i$) in the three different classes of activity (A, B, and C) produces different exercise values ($R_A$, $R_B$, and $R_C$). Different preferred exercise intensities ($S_{p1}$ and $S_{p2}$) can have divergent effects on the exercise value ($R_{p1}$ and $R_{p2}$) of the same sport or between two sports with the same potential exercise value (e.g., bicycling and track running).

cise habits and natural preferences (Borg 1986; figure 12.2). For example, in Sweden and perhaps also in East Asia, most people prefer bicycling as a daily activity, not for training, but to run errands, as a social event, and for psychological relaxation. Most people regard running or jogging as real exercise. Walking is a good exercise but can never be as aerobically demanding as running, unless you use the special technique of a race-walker. Nevertheless, walking for several hours (as during a game of golf) helps you keep fit and burns a lot of calories, but is often underestimated as exercise.

It is recommended that epidemiological determinations of performances of activities of daily life (ADL) assess RPE and integrate these measurements of intensity levels with those of the activity's type, duration, and frequency. A better estimate of the degree of physical activity of individuals thus can be obtained.

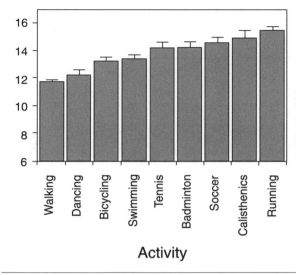

**Figure 12.2** The degree of physical exertion varies for different activities according to RPE ratings by a representative group of Swedish men and women.

# Chapter 13

# Perceived Exertion and Sports

Most RPE studies are performed in laboratories or lablike situations. Real field studies are more unusual, although the use of RPE is common in many sports. Well-designed studies are difficult to carry out in real-life situations and during competitions because the study itself may interfere with the athlete's performance. It may also be rather troublesome to obtain data from a sample that is large enough to allow valid generalizations.

To exercise at an appropriate level, a person has to recognize when that level is reached and how to make suitable changes around that level. This is a very demanding perceptual and psychomotor task. People need reliable measures if they are to monitor exercise intensity effectively. The intensity depends partly, but not mainly, on the chosen sport. Most people find it rather simple and natural to decide what kind of sport to engage in, depending on personal characteristics, abilities, preferences, available facilities, cost,

cultural habits, and social support. How hard to exercise is a more difficult problem. Perceived exertion is one good measure of exercise intensity that can be used in most kinds of sports by both professional and amateur athletes.

The concept of perceived exertion may be seen as having two parts: an active, productive aspect and a more passive, receptive one. The productive aspect refers to the effort and exertion a person consciously intends to apply or is intuitively attempting during a given activity (how much the person wants to tax his or her resources, how hard to make a penalty shot or a tennis serve). The passive aspect of perceived exertion is the strain and fatigue one feels during and after a given activity. For a test on a bicycle ergometer or a treadmill, the instructor sets the speed and resistance, and during a training session the coach sets the tempo. In these situations, a person's freedom to vary the intensity is limited, and thus the passive aspect of perceived exertion is dominant.

## A Brush With Greatness

Many factors have motivated me to work in this field. One of these is my interest in sports. My parents were not great athletes, but my father competed in rifle shooting and had some nice silver cups to show for it. One of my uncles started race-walking when he was 50 years old, and when he was 60, he placed second in a 250-mile, five-day race after the Swedish champion, who was less than half his age. I was the youngest of three brothers who constantly competed in different sports. I was a fairly good athlete but functioned better as a leader, and in 1952 I served as vice president of the Pre-Olympic Games in Stockholm.

When I was elected member and vice chairman of the Swedish Council for Sports Science Research in 1972, one of the physiologists asked me why I had been elected and what sports-related qualifications I had. He decided to test me and asked, "Who beat a world record in Sweden just after World War II, and where and when did it happen?" I immediately answered, "Eskilstuna, 1951, when Rhoden from Jamaica ran 400 m." He looked at me astonished and said, "How did you know that?" "I was running on the outside lane at the time," I answered.

However, during many kinds of sports most people will combine these two aspects. They start with a goal to reach a certain intensity level, for instance, a certain target HR or RPE. They then perceive how hard the exercise actually is and modify it over time.

The different branches of sports can be classified into many categories, depending on technical aspects and psychomotor difficulties involved, how physically and psychologically demanding a branch is, and so on. For applying RPE in sports, I classify sports into five main categories: sports requiring short-term maximal effort, long-term maximal effort, short-term submaximal effort, long-term submaximal effort, and mixed efforts of varying duration.

# Short-Term Maximal Effort

In the first group are sports in which the performance is extremely fast and consists of mainly one maximal effort, for example, a hit or a throw as in shot put. These sports demand good technique and explosive strength. The athlete has to concentrate deeply and make a maximal effort. There is no real variation in effort, and this minimizes the need for subjective scaling to help find the right mental set before the performance. However, after the performance, it may be good to try to estimate how hard the effort actually was, that is, how close to maximum. For maximal-effort sports such as throwing, jumping, or weight lifting, submaximal levels are often used in training to improve and learn the right technique. Thus, in training, perceptual estimates are always useful for identifying appropriate intensity levels.

# Long-Term Maximal Effort

Belonging to the second group are sports that demand a maximal performance that lasts minutes or hours. The athlete has to pace him- or herself perfectly to finish with a maximal achievement, as in most endurance sports such as running a mile or marathon. The performances in this large group of sports are mainly continuous and too long for a maximal effort at the beginning of the activity. Examples of these sports are swimming, running, cross-country skiing, canoeing, and skating.

On the borderline between short-term and long-term performances are those lasting around 30 sec to about 1 1/2 min. A 100-m runner has to run with maximal speed, but a 400-m runner has to pace him- or herself carefully. An athlete running 800 m cannot run as fast as a 400-m runner, but must run faster than a 1,500-m runner. Since an athlete cannot directly monitor the speed after the start, he or she has to rely on the inner clock: the perception of effort and exertion.

A well-trained and experienced athlete must set the appropriate pace from the beginning, then monitor the pace by using feedback from perceived exertion and fatigue. An inexperienced person has great difficulty in setting the right pace. Often in training or test situations an inexperienced person starts too intensely and is then either unable to complete the task or completes it poorly.

Some studies have been done on how athletes are able to monitor appropriate intensity. In chapter 8 a study of a simple running test was presented in which the subjects' task was to set the pace according to a certain perceived intensity. The study showed that trained people are quite able to maintain a constant pace and can do so near a predetermined level. Studies performed on untrained subjects, however, show that without good experience it is rather difficult to set the correct pace. People most often overshoot the speed and then get too tired. This typical pattern of behavior is also a problem with the Cooper 12-min test of aerobic capacity.

A very popular sport in Scandinavian countries is orienteering, in which the athlete runs miles through woods or other terrain to find certain target locations (e.g., a particular big stone or the eastern end of a small pond). This sport is very demanding both physically and mentally. The athlete must run up and down many hills of various sizes, and the exertion is very hard. A scientific study of orienteering recently performed in Sweden by a national coach and exercise physiologists (G. Andersson, personal communication) found HR to be rather stable and to vary less over time than would be expected considering the differences in the terrain. The RPE values recorded at the same time, however, varied much more and followed the actual performance better than HR. There was a great delay or time lag in HR response, which did not change between the harder and the lighter parts of the terrain. The conclusion of the study was that it is better to monitor RPE than HR. Nowadays, many coaches and athletes follow this recommendation in other sports, such as bicycling and cross-country skiing.

Another case in which feelings of perceived exertion can be used is in monitoring the intensity that a runner, cross-country skier, or other endurance athlete chooses for long-distance, low-intensity training, short interval or tempo training, or maximal lactate training. For example, figure 13.1 shows a training program for Swedish cross-country skiers (after Forsberg and Saltin 1988). Athletes must be able to establish an appropriate intensity for the type and duration of their activity.

# Short-Term Submaximal Effort

In the third group are sports in which submaximal effort and exertion are required over a short time. Variation in effort commonly is necessary, as in a kick in football or soccer or a putt in golf.

In this category of sports that demand mainly submaximal effort, there is one group in which the effort should be rather constant, such as bowling or darts, and another group in which the effort has to be varied from very light to very hard, such as basketball (when throwing the ball from different distances), putting in golf, or boccie (boule). The sports that involve great variation of effort and exertion are especially interesting from a perceptual point of view. The athletes must vary the degree of effort needed in a hit or throw (in relation to the differences in distance to the goal). Experienced athletes are extremely well able to intuitively set the right level of intensity. In the old days, an athlete in archery had to rely only on his or her feelings of effort. Now, although there are physical marks on the equipment to rely on, there is still variation of effort during the release.

I don't know of any scientific studies investigating the degree to which it is helpful to consciously identify, visualize, and scale different intensity levels of effort. For a scale to be helpful, one must be well trained in using the scale, and

| | RPE—Intensity | |
|---|---|---|
| | 6   No exertion at all | |
| | 7   Extremely light | |
| | 8 | |
| | 9   Very light | |
| | 10 | |
| Long distance | 11   Light | After about 15 min. |
| | 12 | |
| Short distance | 13   Somewhat hard | |
| | 14 | |
| Short interval | 15   Hard | At the end of intervals/up hills |
| | 16 | |
| Tempo | 17   Very hard | |
| | 18 | |
| "Max" | 19   Extrememly hard | "Lactate" |
| | 20   Maximal exertion | |

**Figure 13.1**   A training model for cross-country skiing with the use of the RPE scale, according to Forsberg (adapted after Forsberg and Saltin 1988).

different perceptual and performance strength levels must be associated with corresponding scale values.

As an example of a research problem, consider the effort necessary for a perfect putt in golf. We could use greens that are level or sloping downhill or uphill with large variations in distance. But before the putt, the golfer has to decide how much effort to use and how long the backswing should be. This is done mainly using intuition, but sometimes people use an "inner voice" with words assigned to the intensity, such as "Now take it very easy" or "This has to be a very hard putt." In situations like this, it is, of course, possible to have the person more consciously and exactly identify the appropriate level using a rating scale. For example, after a close examination the golfer, using the CR10 scale, tells him- or herself, "This has to be a hard putt, a 6" for a rather long uphill putt, or "This must be extremely light (0.5)" for a short downhill putt. This verbalization uses memories and conceptions of muscular effort and performance and facilitates optimal performances. I'm sure it would be possible to learn to do this, but the question is, Would translating the intuitive feeling into a conscious identification improve the golfer's putt shot?

EMG measurements of short-term muscular performances give good information about how muscular activation and relaxation vary over time. In most activities (sports or daily activities of ergonomic interest) it is important that the person know the right activation-relaxation pattern. With a tone generator connected to the EMG apparatus, it is possible to provide auditory feedback for the individual. The person then correlates auditory information with the perception of strain caused by the effort and exertion during the performance. People must learn to identify these inner feelings in order to correct the technique, and people must learn how to exert their strength. It is therefore also important for people to learn to recognize how a good performance feels.

As an example of the importance of learning the right activation-relaxation pattern, we may consider the golf shot. There must be good relaxation before the swing, then a short activation, followed by a very relaxed phase during the backswing, and then a very strong activation when hitting the ball. In a study of the English professional golfer Ian Woosnam, this perfect pattern was found from EMG registration. In less-accomplished golfers some extra muscular activations are often found during the backswing (Janson 1996). There is a great specificity in the muscular activation, and it may be important for the less-accomplished golfer to listen to the sensory signals of muscular strain and learn to synchronize relaxation and activation of the specific muscles. This training may also include psychophysical scaling of the degree of effort and exertion during these sessions. However, the ultimate goal should be for the movement pattern to become so automatic that there is no conscious awareness of the perceived exertion.

# Long-Term Submaximal Effort

Some long-term performances make only submaximal, rather than extreme, demands on muscular strength or endurance capacity. This category includes dance, figure skating, and the rather long, brisk walks in golf. These sports are certainly physically demanding, but the demands on technical knowledge, psychomotor coordination, and mental strength may be still higher.

Most competitive sports do not belong to this category since time for a performance is such an important measurement of excellence (although athletes training for the long-term maximal performances previously described above have to spend most of their training time doing submaximal exercises). To some degree long-term submaximal performance is like going sightseeing for hours without thinking of the time. For the ordinary nonathlete, however, this category includes the most significant part of activities, including brisk walks, jogging, bicycling, hiking, scouting, skating, skiing, swimming, and so on. To be able to monitor and set exercise intensity just right, it is very important to use the perception of exertion (see chapter 11). You want to feel well and to exercise safely so that you don't get too exhausted or hurt yourself.

# Sports With Mixed Efforts of Varying Duration

In this category we find many different sports, including most of the ball sports. The effort may vary from very low to moderate to extremely high or maximal. The performances are not continuous, but consist of intermittent events, often with short pauses. In this group are such sports as tennis, football, soccer, basketball, and handball (as well as golf).

Typical examples are tennis and basketball. You never get as exhausted as in running, but you get much more exhausted than you do playing golf. Most of the time you can run around at a moderate pace, but now and then—such as when you run to the net for a drop shot or back for a lob—you have to make a maximal spurt. You may also sometimes try a maximal explosive movement, as in javelin throwing, when you make your first serve. You have to carefully monitor the intensity for placement and speed of all your ground strokes, volleys, and shifts of pace.

The way an athlete changes his or her effort and pace is very intuitive and from experience. However, some decisions are made more consciously and explicitly, for instance, when serving. A good tactic may be to vary the strength of the serve according to a special program, depending on your own capacity and the opponent's ability. You may tell yourself, "This will be a 90% effort" or "This will be three quarters of maximal." Or you may train yourself with the use of the Borg RPE (or CR10) scale, saying, "This will be a 19" or "This will be 15."

In the 1960s, as a member of the research council for sports in Sweden, I discussed different research projects with active athletes and coaches. I met, among others, Jan-Erik Lundqvist, then the Swedish tennis champion (before Björn Borg). Lundqvist was also American champion, and at his peak he ranked among the three best players in the world. He said that one problem he experienced was how to select an appropriate intensity for a tennis serve. During a long, five-set match a player cannot maintain 100% effort all the time. A player must select a somewhat lower intensity while still maintaining good speed and accuracy. Studying the relationship between effort, exertion, and performance then became one of my projects. The results of a study done in the beginning of the 1970s are shown in figure 13.2.

Figure 13.2 shows that ball speed increases as a rather simple function of effort used in the three groups studied: the Swedish Davis Cup team (male players among the best in the world), male players close to elite, and female players close to elite. As you can see from the figure, only the very best players could really benefit a great deal from 100% effort, with a few players serving up to 200 km/h (55 m/s) without modern racquets. In

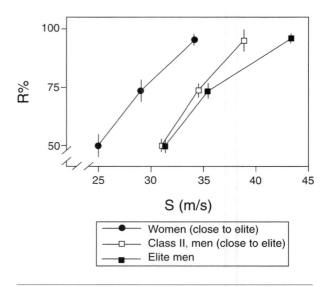

**Figure 13.2** The relationship between subjective effort (R%) and speed of the ball in tennis serve by three groups of players: elite men, men close to the elite level, and women close to the elite level.

order to benefit from maximal effort, psychomotor coordination (the movement pattern or gestalt) has to be close to perfect. Such coordination is something given only to a few people. It would be interesting to see what these S-R functions look like in other sports (e.g., in penalty shots or golf) for people with different techniques and skill.

Sports of special interest are downhill skiing and slalom. To reach a high speed, the skier has to avoid putting too much pressure against the snow. However, sometimes he or she must press very hard to be able to turn or cut down the speed when necessary. This is very strenuous, and the skier must develop a good feeling for the right effort modulation. When the skier gets tired, he or she loses some of that discriminative ability and may perform poorly or even fall. The inexperienced skier when very tired loses control and may increase the speed more than intended. I have named this dramatic course of events "the runaway state." Slalom (or downhill) skiing is one of the few sports, or maybe the only sport, in which you have to use active effort to reduce speed.

A comparison between slalom skiing and cross-country skiing was done by Ceci and coworkers (1986). Data on local perceived exertion (leg exertion) and central perceived exertion (chest, mainly breathlessness) were collected together with HR and blood lactate. Part of the results are shown in figure 13.3.

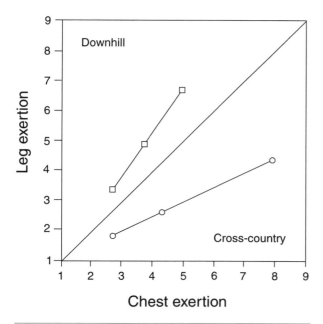

**Figure 13.3** Group means for leg exertion related to chest exertion in cross-country skiing and slalom (Ceci et al. 1986).

The results in the figure agree with common knowledge about the physiological demands for short-duration exercise (see Ceci and Hassmén 1991). In a separate study, data concerning the relationship between RPE and other physiological factors, such as muscle glycogen from the biceps, were also collected. A greatly decreased (50% or more) level of local muscle glycogen was found in several skiers after three days of intensive slalom skiing. The increased leg exertion perceived by these skiers should be a warning signal to slow down and stop for the day to avoid the "runaway" state, which could result in a severe accident.

Another sport of special interest is the biathlon, in which an athlete cross-country skis and at certain locations stops to shoot with a rifle. In this sport the athlete must ski as fast as in ordinary cross-country skiing, but before shooting the athlete must stop and become calm to avoid trembling. In a study in my laboratory we found that the degree of trembling grows with the degree of exercise according to a positively accelerating function with an exponent of the same size as that for perceived exertion. This means that the degree of trembling grows linearly with perceived exertion (Borg and Sjöberg 1981). This knowledge can help biathletes attend to perceived exertion and calm down to an appropriate level before shooting without losing too much time.

A common problem in most sports is rigorous overtraining and stiffness. Many athletes push themselves too much, violating the work-rest principle. In a state of overtraining the athlete experiences mood changes, fatigue, and an elevated perceived exertion during training. A study by O'Connor, Morgan, and Raglin (1991) used the RPE scale during standardized training in swimming (at 90% of $\dot{V}O_2$max). RPE was found to vary, depending on what phase of training the athlete was in. Checking RPE during different types of training may thus be one way (together with other psychological and physiological instruments) to help monitor exercise, choose the right work-rest program, and avoid overtraining.

The ordinary nonathlete has a similar potential for overdoing exercise. In daily activities in the home or garden or during amateur sport activities, it is very important not to strain yourself too much. On the other hand, if you take it too easy, the activity is not meaningful as physical exercise and will not result in the desired fitness. To keep exercise intensity at a level that is just right—in daily life or in sport—you shouldn't work too hard or compete too much, but follow the principle described in chapter 11 and exercise *lagom*—just the right amount.

# References

ACSM. 1991. *Guidelines for exercise testing and prescription*. Philadelphia: Lea & Febiger.

Ahlquist, M.L., and O.G. Franzén. 1994. Encoding of the subjective intensities of sharp dental pain. *Endodontics and Dental Traumatology* 10: 153-66.

Åhsberg, E., and F. Gamberale. 1996. *Upplevd trötthet efter fysiskt arbete. En experimentell utvärdering av ett trötthetsinstrument*. Arbete och Hälsa. Vetenskaplig skriftserie, no. 3. Solna, Sweden: Arbetslivsinstitutet.

Algom, D., and S. Lubel. 1994. Psychophysics in the field: Perception and memory for labor pain. *Perception and Psychophysics* 55: 133-41.

Anand, K.J.S., and C.D. Craig. 1996. New perspectives on the definition of pain. *Pain* 67: 3-6.

Arvidsson, I. 1985. *A study of rehabilitation after knee surgery with special emphasis on pain inhibition on voluntary muscle activation*. Thesis. Stockholm: Karolinska Hospital.

Ashfour, S.S., M.M. Ayoub, A. Mital, and N.J. Bethea. 1983. Perceived exertion of physical effort for various manual handling tasks. *American Industrial Hygiene Association Journal* 44: 223-28.

Asmussen, E. 1979. Muscle fatigue. *Medicine and Science in Sports* 11(4): 313-21.

Åstrand, I. 1960. Aerobic work capacity in men and women with special reference to age. *Acta Physiologica Scandinavica* 169: 1-92

Åstrand, P.-O., and K. Rodahl. 1986. *Textbook of work physiology*. 3rd ed. New York: McGraw-Hill.

Åstrand, P.-O., and B. Saltin. 1961. Oxygen uptake during the first minutes of heavy muscular exercise. *Journal of Applied Physiology* 16: 971-76.

Ayoub, M.M. 1986. Manual materials handling capacity and injury control. In *The perception of exertion in physical work*, ed. by G. Borg and D. Ottoson, 243-53. London: Macmillan.

Bar-Or, O. 1977. Age-related changes in exercise perception. In *Physical work and effort*, ed. by G. Borg, 255-66. Oxford: Pergamon Press.

———. 1987. The Wingate anaerobic test: An update on methodology, reliability and validity. *Sports Medicine* 4: 381-94.

Bar-Or, O., J.S. Skinner, E.R. Buskirk, and G. Borg. 1972. Physiological and perceptual indicators of physical stress in 41- to 60-year-old men who vary in conditioning level and in body fatness. *Medicine and Science in Sports* 2: 96-100.

Bartley, S.H., and E. Chute. 1945. A preliminary clarification of the concept of fatigue. *The Psychological Review* 52: 168-74.

Berglund, B. 1991. Quality assurance in environmental psychophysics. In *Ratio scaling of psychological magnitudes—In honor of the memory of S.S. Stevens*, ed. by S.J. Bolanowski and G.A. Gescheider, 140-62. Hillsdale, NJ: Erlbaum.

Blair, N.S., and J.C. Connolly. 1994. How much physical activity should we do? The case for moderate amounts and intensities of physical activity. In *Moving on: International perspectives on promoting physical activity*, ed. by A.J. Killoran, P. Fentem, and C. Caspersen, 18-34. London: Health Education Authority.

Blomstrand, E., P. Hassmén, S. Andersson, B. Ekblom, and E.A. Newsholme. 1997. Influence of ingesting a solution of branched-chain amino acids on perceived exertion during exercise. *Acta Physiologica Scandinavica* 159: 41-49

Boivie, J., P. Hansson, and U. Lindblom, eds. 1994. *Touch, temperature, and pain in health and disease: Mechanisms and assessments*. Progress in Pain Research and Management, vol. 3. Seattle: IASP Press.

Böje, O. 1944. Energy production, pulmonary ventilation, and length of steps in well-trained runners working on a treadmill. *Acta Physiologica Scandinavica* 7: 362.

Borg, G. 1961a. Interindividual scaling and perception of muscular force. *Kungliga Fysiografiska Sällskapets i Lund Förhandlingar* 12 (31): 117-25.

———. 1961b. Perceived exertion in relation to physical work load and pulse rate. *Kungliga Fysiografiska Sällskapets i Lund Förhandlingar* 11 (31): 105-15.

———. 1961c. *On the perception of speed when car-driving.* Reports from the Department of Psychiatry, no. 3. Umeå, Sweden: Umeå University.

———. 1962a. Physical performance and perceived exertion. *Studia Psychologica et Paedagogica,* Series altera, Investigationes XI. Lund, Sweden: Gleerup.

———. 1962b. A simple rating scale for use in physical work tests. *Kungliga Fysiografiska Sällskapets i Lund Förhandlingar* 2 (32): 7-15.

———. 1964. *On quantitative semantics in connection with psychophysics.* Educational and Psychological Research Bulletin, no. 3. Umeå, Sweden: Umeå University.

———. 1966. *Om bestämning av fysiska "maximalarbeten" och möjligheten att predicera dessa utifrån subjektiv ansträngning.* Rapport från Pedagogisk-Psykologiska Institutionen, no. 6. Umeå, Sweden: Umeå University.

———. 1970a. *Ett enkelt konditionstest för gemene man.* Information från Psykotekniska Institutet, no. 10. Stockholm: University of Stockholm

———. 1970b. Perceived exertion as an indicator of somatic stress. *Scandinavian Journal of Rehabilitation Medicine* 2 (2-3): 92-98.

———. 1972. *A ratio scaling method of interindividual comparisons.* Reports from the Institute of Applied Psychology, no. 27. Stockholm: University of Stockholm.

———. 1973a. *A note on a category scale with "ratio properties" for estimating perceived exertion.* Reports from the Institute of Applied Psychology, no. 36. Stockholm: University of Stockholm.

———. 1973b. *Perceived exertion during walking: A psychophysical function with two additional constants.* Reports from the Institute of Applied Psychology, no. 36. Stockholm: University of Stockholm.

———. 1973c. Perceived exertion: A note on "history" and methods. *Medicine and Science in Sports* 5: 90-93.

———. 1974a. *On a general scale of perceptive intensities.* Reports from the Institute of Applied Psychology, no. 55. Stockholm: University of Stockholm.

———. 1974b. Psychological aspects of physical activities. In *Fitness, health and work capacity. International standards for the assessment,* ed. by L.A. Larson, 141-63. New York: Macmillan.

———, ed. 1977. *Physical work and effort.* Oxford: Pergamon Press.

———. 1978. Subjective effort in relation to physical performance and working capacity. In *Psychology: From research to practice,* ed. by H.L. Pick, Jr., H.W. Liebowitz, J.E. Singer, A. Stenschneider, and H.W. Stevenson, 333-61. New York: Plenum.

———. 1982a. A category scale with ratio properties for intermodal and interindividual comparisons. In *Psychophysical judgement and the process of perception,*

ed. by H.G. Geissler and P. Petzold, 25-34. Berlin: VEB Deutcher Verlag der Wissenschaften.

———. 1982b. Ratings of perceived exertion and heart rates during short-term cycle exercise and their use in a new cycling strength test. *International Journal of Sports Medicine* 3: 153-58.

———. 1985. *An introduction to Borg's RPE-scale.* Ithaca, NY: Mouvement.

———. 1986. Some studies of perceived exertion in sports. In *The perception of exertion in physical work,* ed. by G. Borg and D. Ottoson, 293-302. London: Macmillan.

———. 1990. A general model for interindividual comparison. In *Recent trends in theoretical psychology,* vol. 2, ed. by J.W. Baker, M.E. Hyland, R. van Hezewijk, and S. Terwee, 439-44. New York: Springer-Verlag.

———. 1992. A "fixed star" for the interprocess comparisons. In *Fechner Day 92. Proceedings of the Eighth Annual Meeting of the International Society for Psychophysics,* ed. by G. Borg and G. Neely, 41-45. Stockholm: Stockholm University.

———.1994a. *Borg's RPE scale: A method for measuring perceived exertion.* Stockholm: Borg Perception.

———. 1994b. Psychophysical scaling: An overview. In *Touch, temperature, and pain in health and disease: Mechanisms and assessments,* ed. by J. Boivie, P. Hansson, and U. Lindblom. Progress in Pain Research and Management, vol. 3. Seattle: IASP Press.

Borg, G., and E. Borg. 1991. *A general psychophysical scale of blackness and its possibilities as a test of rating behaviour.* Reports from the Department of Psychology, no. 737. Stockholm: Stockholm University.

———. 1992. *Intelligence and rating behavior in a psychophysical study of size.* Reports from the Department of Psychology, no. 758. Stockholm: Stockholm University.

———. 1994. *Principles and experiments in category-ratio scaling.* Reports from the Department of Psychology, no. 789. Stockholm: Stockholm University.

Borg, G., M. van den Burg, P. Hassmén, L. Kaijser, and S. Tanaka. 1987. Relationships between perceived exertion, HR and HLa in cycling, running, and walking. *Scandinavian Journal of Sports Sciences* 9: 69-77.

Borg, G., and H. Dahlström. 1959. Psykofysisk undersökning av arbete på cykelergometer. *Nordisk Medicin* 62: 1383-86.

———. 1960. The perception of muscular work. *Umeå Vetenskapliga Biblioteks Skriftserie* 5: 3-27.

Borg, G., H. Diamant, L. Ström, and Y. Zotterman. 1967. The relation between neural and perceptual intensity: A comparative study on the neural and psychophysical response to taste stimuli. *Journal of Physiology* 192: 13-20.

Borg, G., M. Domserius, and L. Kaiser. 1990. Effect of alcohol on perceived exertion in relation to heart rate and blood lactate. *European Journal of Applied Psychology* 60: 382-84.

Borg, G., B. Edgren, and D. Levin. 1978. *Idrott och motion, ansträngning och motivation. Del. 1 Vilka motionerar och varför? Hur och med vilken intensitet.* Information från Psykotekniska Institutet, no. 101. Stockholm: University of Stockholm.

Borg, G., B. Edgren, and G. Marklund. 1971. *A simple walk test of physical work capacity.* Reports from the Institute of Applied Psychology, no. 18. Stockholm: University of Stockholm.

————. 1973. *The reliability and stability of the indicators in a simple walk test.* Reports from the Institute of Applied Psychology, no. 35. Stockholm: University of Stockholm.

Borg, G., C.-G. Edström, H. Linderholm, and G. Marklund. 1972. Changes in physical performance induced by amphetamine and amobarbital. *Psychopharmacologia* 26: 10-18.

Borg, G., C.-G. Edström, and G. Marklund. 1970. *A new method to determine the exponent for perceived force in physical work.* Reports from the Institute of Applied Psychology, no. 4. Stockholm: University of Stockholm.

Borg, G., A. Herbert, and R. Ceci. 1984. *Some characteristics of a simple run test and its correlation with a bicycle ergometer test of physical working capacity.* Reports from the Department of Psychology, no. 625. Stockholm: Stockholm University.

Borg, G., A. Holmgren, and I. Lindblad. 1981. Quantitative evaluation of chest pain. *Acta Medica Scandinavica* 644 (suppl.): 43-45.

Borg, G., and J. Hosman. 1970. *The metric properties of adverbs.* Reports from the Institute of Applied Psychology, no. 7. Stockholm: University of Stockholm.

Borg, G., and S.-E. Johansson. 1986. The growth of perceived exertion during a prolonged bicycle ergometer test at a constant work load. In *The perception of exertion in physical work,* ed. by G. Borg and D. Ottoson, 47-55. London: Macmillan.

Borg, G., J.-G. Karlsson, and L.-G. Ekelund. 1977. A comparison between two work tests controlled subjectively and by heart-rate. In *Physical work and effort,* ed. by G. Borg, 239-54. New York: Pergamon Press.

Borg, G., J.-G. Karlsson, and I. Lindblad. 1976. *Quantitative variation of subjective symptoms during ergometer work.* Reports from the Institute of Applied Psychology, no. 72. Stockholm: University of Stockholm.

Borg, G., and I. Lindblad. 1976. *The determination of subjective intensities in verbal descriptors of symptoms.* Reports from the Institute of Applied Psychology, no. 75. Stockholm: University of Stockholm.

Borg, G., and H. Linderholm. 1967. Perceived exertion and pulse rate during graded exercise in various age groups. *Exerptum. Acta Medica Scandinavica* 472 (suppl.): 194-204.

————. 1970. Exercise performance and perceived exertion in patients with coronary insufficiency, arterial hypertension and vasoregulatory asthenia. *Acta Medica Scandinavica* 187: 17-26.

Borg, G., G. Ljunggren, and R. Ceci. 1985. The increase of perceived exertion, aches and pain in the legs, heart rate and blood lactate during exercise on a bicycle ergometer. *European Journal of Applied Physiology* 54: 343-49.

Borg, G., G. Ljunggren, and L.E. Marks. 1985. *General and differential aspects of perceived exertion and loudness assessed by two new methods.* Reports from the Department of Psychology, no. 636. Stockholm: Stockholm University.

Borg, G., and B.J. Noble. 1974. Perceived exertion. In *Exercise and sport science reviews,* ed. by J. Wilmore, 131-53. New York: Academic Press.

Borg, G., and B. Nordheden. 1976. *A further study on the effects of the rate of work load increase on muscular performance on bicycle ergometer.* Reports from the Institute of Applied Psychology, no. 74. Stockholm: University of Stockholm.

Borg, G., and M. Ohlsson. 1975. *A study of two variants of a simple run-test for determining physical working capacity.* Reports from the Institute of Applied Psychology, no. 61. Stockholm: University of Stockholm.

Borg. G., and D. Ottoson, eds. 1986. *The perception of exertion in physical work.* London: Macmillan.

Borg, G., M.A. Sherman, and B.J. Noble. 1968. Paper presented at the annual meeting of the ACSM, held at State College, Pennsylvania, May.

Borg, G., and H. Sjöberg. 1981. The variation of hand steadiness with physical stress. *Journal of Motor Behavior* 13: 110-16.

Capodaglio, P., and E.M. Capodaglio. 1995. Ratings of perceived exertion in exercise prescription. *Europa Mediophysica* 31: 95-105.

Capodaglio, P., E.M. Capodaglio, and G. Bazzini. 1995. Tolerability to prolonged lifting tasks assessed by subjective perception and physiological responses. *Ergonomics* 38: 2118-28.

Ceci, R., G. Borg, P. Borg, and S.-E. Johansson. 1986. Perceived exertion, heart rate and blood lactate in downhill skiing as compared to cross-country—A pilot study. In *The perception of exertion in physical work,* ed. by G. Borg and D. Ottoson, 293-302. London: Macmillan.

Ceci, R., and P. Hassmén. 1991. Self-monitored exercise at three different RPE-intensities in treadmill versus field running. *Medicine and Science in Sports and Exercise* 23: 732-38.

Cooper, K.H. 1968. A means of assessing maximum oxygen intake. *Journal of the American Medical Association* 203: 201-4.

Coren, S, L.M. Ward, and J.T. Enns. 1994. *Sensation and perception.* 4th ed. New York: Harcourt Brace Jovanovich.

Costa, P.T., and T.A. Widiger, Jr., eds. 1994. *Personality disorders and the five-factor model of personality.* Washington, DC: American Psychological Association.

Dishman, R.K., R.E. Graham, R.G. Holly, and J.G. Tieman. 1991. Estimates of type A behavior do not predict exertion during graded exercise. *Medicine and Science in Sports and Exercise* 11: 1276-82.

Dray, A., L. Urban, and A. Dickenson. 1994. Pharmacology of chronic pain. *Trends in Pharmacological Sciences* 15 (6): 190-97.

Edgren, B., and G. Borg. 1975. *The reliability and stability of the indicators in a simple run test.* Reports from the Institute of Applied Psychology, no. 57. Stockholm: University of Stockholm.

Edgren, B., G. Marklund., L.-O. Nordesjö, and G. Borg. 1976. The validity of four bicycle ergometer tests. *Medicine and Science in Sports* 8: 179-85.

Eisler, H. 1962. Subjective scale of force for a large muscle group. *Journal of Experimental Psychology* 64: 253-57.

Eisler, H., and E.E. Roskam. 1977. Multidimensional similarity: An experimental and theoretical comparison of vector, distance, and set theoretical models: II. Multidimensional analyses: The subjective space. *Acta Psychologica* 41 (5): 335-63.

Ekblom, B., and A.N. Goldberg. 1971. The influence of physical training and other factors on the subjective rating of perceived exertion. *Acta Physiologica Scandinavica* 83: 399-406.

Ekman, G., B. Hosman, R. Lindman, L. Ljungberg, and C.A. Åkesson. 1968. Interindividual differences in scaling performance. *Perceptual and Motor Skills* 26: 815-23.

Ellermeier, W., W. Westphal, and M. Heidenfelder. 1991. On the "absoluteness" of category and magnitude scales of pain. *Perception and Psychophysics* 49: 159-66.

Eston, R.G., and J.G. Williams. 1988. Reliability of ratings of perceived effort for regulation of exercise intensity. *British Journal of Sports Medicine* 22: 153-54.

Eysenck, H.J. 1994. Trait theories in personality. In *Companion encyclopedia of personality,* ed. by A.M. Coolman, 622-40. London: Routledge.

Falmagne, J.-C. 1985. *Elements of psychophysical theory.* New York: Oxford University Press.

Fechner, G.T. 1860. *Elemente der Psychophysik.* Leipzig, Germany: Breitkopf & Härtel.

Fleishman, E.A., D.L. Gebbart, and J.C. Hogan. 1986. The perception of physical effort in job tasks. In *The perception of exertion in physical work,* ed. by G. Borg and D. Ottoson, 225-42. London: Macmillan.

Forsberg, A., and B. Saltin. 1988. *Konditionsträning.* Stockholm: Idrottens forskningsråd, Sveriges Riksidrottsförbund.

Franzén, O.G., and M.L. Ahlquist. 1989. The intensive aspect of information processing in the intradental A-delta system in man: A psychophysiological analysis of sharp dental pain. *Behavioral Brain Research* 33: 1-11.

Gamberale, F. 1990. Perception of effort in manual materials handling. *Scandinavian Journal of Work, Environment & Health* 16: 59-66.

Gamberale, F., and I. Holmér. 1977. Heart rate and perceived exertion in simulated work with high heat stress. In *Physical work and effort,* ed. by G. Borg, 323-32. New York: Pergamon Press.

Gesheider, G.A. 1985. *Psychophysics: Method, theory, and application.* Hillsdale, NJ: Erlbaum.

Gibson, J.J. 1979. *The ecological approach to visual perception.* Boston: Houghton Mifflin.

Gracely, R.H. 1979. Psychophysical assessment of human pain. *Advances in Pain Research and Therapy* 3: 805-24.

Gracely, R.H., and R. Dubner. 1981. Pain assessment in humans—A reply to Hall. *Pain* 11: 109-20.

Gracely, R.H., R. Dubner, P. McGrath, and M. Heft. 1978. New methods of pain measurement and their application to pain control. *International Dental Journal* 28: 52-65.

Grosse-Lordemann, H., and E.A. Müller. 1937. Der Einfluss der Leistung unter der Arbeitsgeschwindigkeit auf das Arbeitsmaximum und den Wirkungsgrad beim Radfahren. *Arbeitsphysiologie* 9: 454-75.

Guilford, J.P. 1954. *Psychometric methods.* New York: McGraw-Hill.

Gutman, M.C., R.W. Squires, M.L. Pollock, C. Foster, and J. Anholm. 1981. Perceived exertion–heart rate relationship during exercise testing and training in cardiac patients. *Journal of Cardiac Rehabilitation* 1: 52-59.

Hage, P. 1981. Perceived exertion: One measure of exercise intensity. *The Physician and Sportsmedicine* 9: 136-43.

Hagen, K.B. 1994. *Physical work load and perceived exertion during forest work and experimental repetitive lifting. With special reference to lifting technique.* Thesis. Stockholm: Karolinska Institute.

Halverson, C.F., Jr., G.A. Kohnstamm, and R.P. Martin, eds. 1994. *The developing structure of temperament and personality from infancy to adulthood.* Hillsdale, NJ: Erlbaum.

Harms-Ringdahl, K. 1986. On assessment of shoulder exercise and load-elicited pain in the cervical spine. Biomechanical analysis of load-EMG-methodological studies of pain provoked by extreme position. Thesis. Stockholm: Karolinska Institute. *Scandinavian Journal of Rehabilitation Medicine* 18 (suppl. 14).

Harms-Ringdahl, K., H. Brodin, L. Eklund, and G. Borg. 1983. Discomfort and pain from loaded passive joint structures. *Scandinavian Journal of Rehabilitation Medicine* 15: 205-11.

Harms-Ringdahl, K., A.M. Carlsson, J. Ekholm, A. Raustorp, T. Svensson, and H.-G. Toresson. 1986. Pain assessment with different intensity scales in response to loading of joint structures. *Pain* 27: 401-11.

Hassmén, P., and R. Ceci. 1990. *Indicators of aerobic capacity: The relation between an outdoor run test and a conventional cycle ergometer test in a group of females.* Reports from the Department of Psychology, no. 713. Stockholm: Stockholm University.

Hassmén, P., R. Ståhl, and G. Borg. 1993. Psychophysiological responses to exercise in type A/B men. *Psychosomatic Medicine* 55: 178-84.

Holzmann, P. 1982. ARBAN—A new method for analyses of ergonomic effort. *Applied Ergonomics* 13: 82-86.

Hueting, J.E. 1965. An attempt to quantify sensations of general physical fatigue. *Proceedings of the 1st International Psychology of Sport*, Rome.

International Organization for Standardization. 1981. *Ergonomic principles in the design of work systems*, part 4.2. ISO 6385.

Janson, L. 1996. Avspänd teknik. Fyfiska och psykologiska aspekter i kombination. *Svensk Idrottsforskning* 1: 31-33.

Johansson, S.-E., and G. Borg. 1993. Perception of heavy work operations by tank truck drivers. *Applied Ergonomics* 24: 421-26.

Johansson S.-E., and G. Ljunggren. 1989. Perceived exertion during a self-imposed pace of work for a group of cleaners. *Applied Ergonomics* 20 (4): 307-12.

Jones, F.N., and M.J. Marcus. 1961. The subject effect in judgments of subjective magnitude. *Journal of Experimental Psychology* 61: 40-44.

Karvonen, M., K. Kentala, and O. Musta. 1957. The effect of training heart rate: A longitudinal study. *Annales Medicinae Experiemenales et Biolpgiae Fenniae* 35: 307-15.

Kinsman, R.A., and P.C. Weiser. 1975. Subjective symptomatology during work and fatigue. In *Psychological aspects and physiological correlates of work and fatigue*, ed. by E. Simonson and P.C. Weiser, 336-405. Springfield, IL: Charles C Thomas.

Komi, P.V., and S.-L. Karppi. 1977. Genetic and environmental variation in perceived exertion and heart rate during bicycle ergometer work. In *Physical work and effort*, ed. by G. Borg, 91-100. New York: Pergamon Press.

Lamb, K.L. 1995. Children's ratings of effort during cycle ergometry: An examination of the validity of two effort scales. *Pediatric Exercise Science* 7 (4): 407-21.

Lindblom, U. 1987. Om smärta. *Läkartidningen* 84: 2472.

Ljunggren, G. 1985. *Studies of perceived exertion during bicycle ergometer exercise—Some applications*. Thesis. Stockholm: Stockholm University.

———. 1986. Observer ratings of perceived exertion in relation to self ratings and heart rate. *Applied Ergonomics* 17 (2): 117-25.

Ljunggren, G., and S.-E. Johansson. 1988. Use of submaximal measures of perceived exertion during bicycle ergometer exercise as predictor of maximal work capacity. *Journal of Sports Sciences* 6: 189-203.

Mahon, A., and M. Marsh. 1992. Reliability of the rating of perceived exertion at ventilatory threshold in children. *International Journal of Sports Medicine* 13: 567-71.

Marks, L.E., G. Borg, and G. Ljunggren. 1983. Individual differences in perceived exertion assessed by two new methods. *Perception and Psychophysics* 34: 280-88.

McNemar, Q. 1957. *Psychological statistics*. 2nd ed. New York: Wiley.

Merskey, H. 1991. The definition of pain. *European Journal of Psychiatry* 6: 153-59.

Merskey, H., and N. Bogduk. 1994. *Classification of chronic pain: Description of chronic pain syndromes and definitions of pain terms*. Seattle: IASP Press.

Miyashita, M., K. Onodera, and I. Tabata. 1986. How Borg's RPE-scale has been applied to Japanese. In *The perception of exertion in physical work*, ed. by G. Borg and D. Ottoson, 27-34. London: Macmillan.

Morgan, W.P. 1973. Psychological factors influencing perceived exertion. *Medicine and Science in Sports* 5: 97-103.

Morgan, W.P., and G. Borg. 1977. Perception of effort in the prescription of physical activity. In *The humanistic and mental health aspects of sports exercise and recreation*, ed. by T.T. Craig, 126-29. Chicago: American Medical Association.

Morgan, W.P., and M.L. Pollock. 1977. Psychologic characterization of the elite distance runner. *Annals of the New York Academy of Sciences* 301: 382-403.

Morris, W. 1969. *The American Heritage dictionary of the English language*. New York: American Heritage.

Mountcastle, V.B., G.F. Poggio, and G. Werner. 1963. The relation of thalamic cell response to peripheral stimuli varied over an intensive continuum. *Journal of Neurophysiology* 26: 807-34.

Müller, F., G. Neely, and E. Fichtl. 1995. Scaling of loudness, perceived exertion, and pain intensity: A comparison between the category-partitioning (CP) and category ratio (CR-20) scaling procedures. In *Category-ratio scaling of sensory magnitude in comparison with other methods*, by G. Neely (thesis). Stockholm: Stockholm University.

Neely, G. 1995. *Category-ratio scaling of sensory magnitude in comparison with other methods*. Thesis. Stockholm: Stockholm University.

Neely, G., G. Ljunggren, C. Sylvén, and G. Borg. 1992. Comparison between the visual analogue scale (VAS) and the category ratio scale (CR-10) for the evaluation of leg exertion. *International Journal of Sports Medicine* 13: 133-36.

Noble, B.J., and G. Borg. 1972. Perceived exertion during walking and running. In *Proceedings of the 17th International Congress of Applied Psychology*, ed. by R. Piret, 387-92. Brussels.

Noble, B., G. Borg, R. Ceci, I. Jacobs, and P. Kaiser. 1983. A category-ratio perceived exertion scale: Relationship to blood and muscle lactates and heart rate. *Medicine and Science in Sports and Exercise* 15: 523-28.

Noble, B. and R. Robertson. 1996. *Perceived exertion*. Champaign, IL: Human Kinetics.

O'Connor, P.J., W.P. Morgan, and J.S. Raglin. 1991. Psychobiologic effects of 3 days of increased training in female and male swimmers. *Medicine and Science in Sports and Exercise* 23: 1055-61.

Onions, C.T., ed. 1968. *The Shorter Oxford English Dictionary*. 3rd ed., prepared by W. Little, H.W. Fowler, and J. Coulson. London: Oxford University Press.

Pandolf, K.B. 1975. Psychological and physiological factors influencing perceived exertion. In *Physical work and effort,* ed. by G. Borg, 371-83. New York: Pergamon Press.

———. 1983. Advances in the study and application of perceived exertion. *Exercise and Sport Sciences Reviews* 11: 118-58.

Pandolf, K.B., R.L. Burse, and R.F. Goldman. 1975. Differentiated ratings of perceived exertion during physical conditioning for older individuals using leg-weight loading. *Perceptual and Motor Skills* 40: 563-74.

Pavlina, Z., and I. Saric. 1975. *The interrelationship among three measurements of physical stress: Absolute heart rate, relative heart rate and ratings of perceived effort.* Reports from the Department of Psychology, no. 56. Stockholm: Stockholm University.

Poffenberger, H.T. 1928. Effects of continuous work upon output and feelings. *Journal of Applied Psychology* 12: 459-67.

Pollock, M., A. Jackson, and C. Foster. 1986. The use of the perception scale for exercise prescription. In *The perception of exertion in physical work,* ed. by G. Borg and D. Ottoson, 161-78. London: Macmillan.

Price, D.D. 1988. *Psychological and neural mechanisms of pain.* New York: Raven Press.

———. 1994. On pain measurements. In *Touch, temperature, and pain in health and disease: Mechanisms and assessments,* ed. by J. Boivie, P. Hansson, and U. Lindblom. Progress in Pain Research and Management, vol. 3. Seattle: IASP Press.

Price, D.D., P.A. McGrath, A. Rafii, and B. Buckingham. 1983. The validation of visual analogue scales as ratio scale measures for chronic and experimental pain. *Pain* 17: 45-56.

Quine, W.V. 1987. *Quiddities.* Cambridge: Harvard University Press.

———. 1990. *Pursuit of truth.* Cambridge: Harvard University Press.

Rejeski, W.J. 1985. Perceived exertion: An active or passive process? *Journal of Sport Psychology* 7: 371-78.

Robertson, R.J., R.L. Gillespie, J. McCarthy, and K.D Rose. 1979. Differentiated perceptions of exertion: Part II. Relationship to local and central physiological responses. *Perceptual and Motor Skills* 49: 691-97.

Rollman, G.B. 1977. Signal detection theory measurement of pain: A review and critique. *Pain* 3: 187-211.

Runesson, S., and G. Frykholm. 1981. Visual perception of lifted weight. *Journal of Experimental Psychology: Human Perception and Performance* 7: 733-40.

Sagal, P., and G. Borg. 1993. The range principle and the problem of other minds. *British Journal for the Philosophy of Science* 44: 477-91.

Sjöstrand, T. 1947. Changes in respiratory organs of workmen at an ore smelting works. *Acta Medica Scandinavica* 196 (suppl.): 687-99.

Skinner, J.S., R. Hutsler, V. Bergsteinova, and E.R. Buskirk. 1973. The validity and reliability of a rating scale of perceived exertion. *Medicine and Science in Sports* 5: 94-96.

Spielberger, C.D. 1975. Anxiety: State-trait process. In *Stress and Anxiety,* vol. 1, ed. by C.D. Spielberger and I.G. Sarason. Washington, DC: Hemisphere.

Stamford, B.A. 1976. Validity and reliability of subjective ratings of perceived exertion during work. *Ergonomics* 19: 53-60.

Stevens, J.C., and J.D. Mach. 1959. Scales of apparent force. *Journal of Experimental Psychology* 58: 405-13.

Stevens, J.C., and L.E. Marks. 1980. Cross-modality matching functions generated by magnitude estimation. *Perception and Psychophysics* 27: 379-89.

Stevens, S.S. 1957. On the psychophysical law. *The Psychological Review* 64: 153-81.

———. 1971. Issues in psychophysiological measurement. *The Psychological Review* 78: 426-50.

———. 1975. *Psychophysics: Introduction to its perceptual, neural, and social prospects.* New York: Wiley.

Stevens, S.S., and E.H. Galanter. 1957. Ratio scales and category scales for a dozen perceptual continua. *Journal of Experimental Psychology* 54: 377-411.

Swedborg, I., G. Borg, and M. Sarnelid. 1981. Somatic sensation and discomfort in the arm of post-mastectomy patients. *Scandinavian Journal of Rehabilitation and Medicine* 13: 23-29.

Sylvén, C., G. Borg, R. Brandt, B. Beerman, and B. Jonzon. 1988. Dose-effect relationship of adenosine provoked angina pectoris–like pain—A study of the psychosocial power function. *European Heart Journal* 9: 87-91.

Tornvall, G. 1963. Assessment of physical capabilities. *Acta Physiologica Scandinavica* 201 (suppl.): 53.

Turk, D.C., and R. Melzack, eds. 1992. *Handbook of pain assessment.* New York: Guilford Press.

Ulmer, H.-V., U. Janz, and H. Löllgen. 1977. Aspects of the validity of Borg's scale. Is it measuring stress or strain? In *Physical work and effort,* ed. by G. Borg, 181-96. Oxford: Pergamon Press.

Vernon, M.D. 1962. *A further study of visual perception.* London: Cambridge University Press.

Warren, R.M. 1981. Measurement of sensory intensity. *The Behavioral and Brain Sciences* 4: 175-223.

Weiser, P.C., and D.A. Stamper. 1977. Psychophysiological interactions leading to increased effort, leg fatigue, and respiratory distress during prolonged, strenuous bicycle riding. In *Physical work and effort,* ed. by G. Borg, 410-16. Oxford: Pergamon Press.

Wilmore, J.H., F.B. Roby, P.R. Stanforth, M.J. Buono, S.H. Constable, U. Tsao, and B.J. Lowdon. 1986. Ratings of perceived exertion, heart rate, and power output in predicting maximal oxygen uptake during submaximal cycle ergometry. *The Physician and Sportsmedicine* 14: 133-43.

Wos, H., T. Marek, C. Noworol, and G. Borg. 1988. The reliability of self-ratings based on Borg's scale for hand-arm vibrations of short duration: Part II. *International Journal of Industrial Ergonomics* 2: 151-56.

Zwislocki, J.J., and D.A. Goodman. 1980. Absolute scaling of sensory magnitude: A validation. *Perception & Psychophysics* 28: 28-38.

# Index

# About the Author

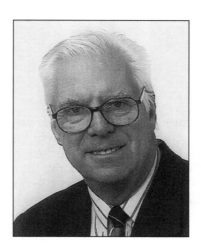

Gunnar Borg, PhD, introduced the field of perceived exertion during the latter part of the 1950s. Since then, he has won international renown for his work in developing methods for measuring perceived exertion and pain. His method for measuring perceived exertion is the main method used in the field, and his new scale, the Borg CR10 scale, is used for measuring both perceived exertion and pain, and other subjective magnitudes.

He is the author of *Physical Performance and Perceived Exertion*, the book that introduced the field of perception. He also is coauthor of "The relation between neural and perceptual intensity: A comparative study on the neural and psychophysical response to taste stimuli," published in the *Journal of Physiology* in 1967. The article is fundamental to the science of psychophysiology. It marked the first time that perceptual magnitudes could be correlated directly to afferent neurophysiological responses of human beings. Another fundamental contribution is Borg's Range Model, which provides basic principles for determinations of "absolute" levels of intensity and how inter-individual and intermodal comparisons can be done.

Borg has organized and served as chair for numerous international symposia in the field of perception. He lectures worldwide, particularly in the United States, Canada, and Japan. He was nominated for the Australian Prize by the American College of Sports Medicine for research in the field of perception with applications for the benefit of mankind.

Currently professor emeritus of perception and psychophysics at Stockholm University, Borg's educational background encompasses the fields of psychology, philosophy, education, physiology, and sports. Borg was an associate professor at the Medical School in Umea, Sweden, from 1962 to 1968, during which time he also served as director of the laboratory for clinical psychology at the Umea Hospital. He was professor of perception and psychophysics at Stockholm University from 1987 to 1994.

Borg was elected a member of the Royal Swedish Academy for Engineering Sciences in 1970. The following year, the King of Sweden awarded Borg the title of Professor. Borg is a member of the International Association of Applied Psychology, the International Association for the Study of Pain, and the International Society for Psychophysics.

Borg and his wife Yvonne live in Rimbo, Sweden. His leisure activities include tennis, golf, skiing, and "walk-and-talk."

# *Appendix*

## Scales and Instructions

A detailed account of how the scales should be administered is given in chapter 7. Everyone who wants to use the scales should read that chapter carefully. The test leader must devote adequate time to explain the purpose of the test, what the subject is going to rate, how it is going to be done, and so forth. The subject must understand that it is his or her perception or subjective feeling that he or she shall attend to—and not the physical task or the psychological cues. It is the inner feeling as a subjective phenomenon that is important and that should be the focus.

The test leader should read the instructions together with the subject and show the scale. The subject may be given the scale together with the instruction while waiting for the examination. It is important that the subject has enough time to look at the scale and get acquainted with the expressions and the range of numbers. The test leader still has the responsibility to show the scale and explain its administration.

Sometimes special material for instructing, training, and testing the subject may be needed: this is often good to have in order to improve the understanding of the scale and it's use, as well as for studying individual rating behavior. The RPE scale is simpler in construction than the CR10 scale. And most often no special training material is necessary for it. The CR10 scale is a bit more complicated, however, and it is therefore good to use special test material for rating behavior or some short questions such as those given in chapter 7.

Scaling pain is often also more difficult than scaling perceived exertion As a concept and as an empirical variable, perceived exertion is rather simple; it refers to heavy physical work of a similar kind, such as running, bicycling, or lifting heavy objects over a period of time.

Pain, on the other hand, may refer to many different kinds of sensations and emotions and is not so simple to scale. People also differ quite a lot in their previous experiences of pain. They may use different personal anchors, referring to memories of something actually perceived or to something imagined or "extrapolated" (e.g., from something seen or heard about). Therefore the instruction has to be rather detailed, and it's good to use special examples. When determining what personal anchors to use as 10 on the scale, the subjects should describe their previous experiences of pain and then scale them, using their conceptions of maximal perceived exertion as an anchor. After having done that and getting numbers, such as 12 for a terrible toothache and 13 for a kidney stone attack or child birth, it is possible to pick their memory and conception of their previous worst pain and use that as a personal anchor. That will then be their "max P" and set to 10. It is also possible to go on and use the Max Perceived Exertion as 10. What anchor used in a special study or examination must, of course, be noted.

It is vitally important that the subject understand what the anchor is and that 10 is the main point of reference denoted "max P" ("P" refers to a perception, such as perceived exertion or pain. It may also stand for other perceptions, emotions or conceptions). What kinds of perceptions or attributes "max P" stands for must be explained very clearly, as must what we want the subject to rate. In a clinical stress test with an ergometer it is often of great diagnostic value to get ratings of breathlessness, strain, and fatigue in the working muscles and / or joints, as well as chest (heart) pain and other symptoms (e.g., feeling sick).

The test leader must never forget to ask the subject if he or she has any questions!

| | |
|---|---|
| 6 | No exertion at all |
| 7 | |
| | Extremely light |
| 8 | |
| 9 | Very light |
| 10 | |
| 11 | Light |
| 12 | |
| 13 | Somewhat hard |
| 14 | |
| 15 | Hard   (heavy) |
| 16 | |
| 17 | Very hard |
| 18 | |
| 19 | Extremely hard |
| 20 | Maximal exertion |

# Borg's RPE Scale Instructions

While exercising we want you to rate your perception of exertion, i.e., how heavy and strenuous the exercise feels to you. The perception of exertion depends mainly on the strain and fatigue in your muscles and on your feeling of breathlessness or aches in the chest.

Look at this rating scale; we want you to use this scale from 6 to 20, where 6 means "no exertion at all" and 20 means "maximal exertion."

9     corresponds to "very light" exercise. For a normal, healthy person it is like walking slowly at his or her own pace for some minutes.

13     on the scale is "somewhat hard" exercise, but it still feels OK to continue.

17     "very hard" is very strenuous. A healthy person can still go on, but he or she really has to push him- or herself. It feels very heavy, and the person is very tired.

19     on the scale is an extremely strenuous exercise level. For most people this is the most strenuous exercise they have ever experienced.

Try to appraise your feeling of exertion as honestly as possible, without thinking about what the actual physical load is. Don't underestimate it, but don't overestimate it either. It's your own feeling of effort and exertion that's important, not how it compares to other people's. What other people think is not important either. Look at the scale and the expressions and then give a number.

Any questions?

| | |
|---|---|
| 6 | No exertion at all |
| 7 | |
| 8 | Extremely light |
| 9 | Very light |
| 10 | |
| 11 | Light |
| 12 | |
| 13 | Somewhat hard |
| 14 | |
| 15 | Hard   (heavy) |
| 16 | |
| 17 | Very hard |
| 18 | |
| 19 | Extremely hard |
| 20 | Maximal exertion |

Borg RPE scale
© Gunnar Borg, 1970, 1985, 1984, 1998

| | |
|---|---|
| 6 | No exertion at all |
| 7 | |
| 8 | Extremely light |
| 9 | Very light |
| 10 | |
| 11 | Light |
| 12 | |
| 13 | Somewhat hard |
| 14 | |
| 15 | Hard   (heavy) |
| 16 | |
| 17 | Very hard |
| 18 | |
| 19 | Extremely hard |
| 20 | Maximal exertion |

Borg RPE scale
© Gunnar Borg, 1970, 1985, 1984, 1998

## Borg's RPE Scale Instructions

While exercising we want you to rate your perception of exertion, i.e., how heavy and strenuous the exercise feels to you. The perception of exertion depends mainly on the strain and fatigue in your muscles and on your feeling of breathlessness or aches in the chest.

Look at this rating scale; we want you to use this scale from 6 to 20, where 6 means "no exertion at all" and 20 means "maximal exertion."

9  corresponds to "very light" exercise. For a normal, healthy person it is like walking slowly at his or her own pace for some minutes.

13  on the scale is "somewhat hard" exercise, but it still feels OK to continue.

17  "very hard" is very strenuous. A healthy person can still go on, but he or she really has to push him- or herself. It feels very heavy, and the person is very tired.

19  on the scale is an extremely strenuous exercise level. For most people this is the most strenuous exercise they have ever experienced.

Try to appraise your feeling of exertion as honestly as possible, without thinking about what the actual physical load is. Don't underestimate it, but don't overestimate it either. It's your own feeling of effort and exertion that's important, not how it compares to other people's. What other people think is not important either. Look at the scale and the expressions and then give a number.
Any questions?

## Borg's RPE Scale Instructions

While exercising we want you to rate your perception of exertion, i.e., how heavy and strenuous the exercise feels to you. The perception of exertion depends mainly on the strain and fatigue in your muscles and on your feeling of breathlessness or aches in the chest.

Look at this rating scale; we want you to use this scale from 6 to 20, where 6 means "no exertion at all" and 20 means "maximal exertion."

9  corresponds to "very light" exercise. For a normal, healthy person it is like walking slowly at his or her own pace for some minutes.

13  on the scale is "somewhat hard" exercise, but it still feels OK to continue.

17  "very hard" is very strenuous. A healthy person can still go on, but he or she really has to push him- or herself. It feels very heavy, and the person is very tired.

19  on the scale is an extremely strenuous exercise level. For most people this is the most strenuous exercise they have ever experienced.

Try to appraise your feeling of exertion as honestly as possible, without thinking about what the actual physical load is. Don't underestimate it, but don't overestimate it either. It's your own feeling of effort and exertion that's important, not how it compares to other people's. What other people think is not important either. Look at the scale and the expressions and then give a number.
Any questions?

| | | |
|---|---|---|
| 0 | Nothing at all | "No P" |
| 0.3 | | |
| 0.5 | Extremely weak | Just noticeable |
| 1 | Very weak | |
| 1.5 | | |
| 2 | Weak | Light |
| 2.5 | | |
| 3 | Moderate | |
| 4 | | |
| 5 | Strong | Heavy |
| 6 | | |
| 7 | Very strong | |
| 8 | | |
| 9 | | |
| **10** | **Extremely strong** | **"Max P"** |
| 11 | | |
| ⌇ | | |
| ● | Absolute maximum | Highest possible |

Borg CR10 scale
© Gunnar Borg, 1981, 1982, 1998

# Borg's CR10 Scale Instructions

**Basic instruction**: 10, "Extremely strong—Max P," is the main anchor. It is the strongest perception (P) you have ever experienced. It may be possible, however, to experience or to imagine something even stronger. Therefore, "Absolute maximum" is placed somewhat further down the scale without a fixed number and marked with a dot "•". If you perceive an intensity stronger than 10, you may use a higher number.

Start with a *verbal expression* and then choose a *number*. If your perception is "Very weak," say 1; if "Moderate," say 3; and so on. You are welcome to use half values (such as 1.5, or 3.5 or decimals, for example, 0.3, 0.8, or 2.3). It is very important that you answer what *you* perceive and not what you believe you ought to answer. Be as honest as possible and try not to overestimate or underestimate the intensities.

**Scaling perceived exertion**: We want you to rate your perceived (P) exertion, that is, how heavy and strenuous the exercise feels to you. This depends mainly on the strain and fatigue in your muscles and on your feeling of breathlessness or aches in the chest. But you must only attend to your subjective feelings and not to the physiological cues or what the actual physical load is.

1   is "very light" like walking slowly at your own pace for several minutes.

3   is not especially hard; it feels fine, and it is no problem to continue.

5   you are tired, but you don't have any great difficulties

7   you can still go on but have to push yourself very much. You are very tired.

10   This is as hard as most people have ever experienced before in their lives.

•   This is "Absolute maximum," for example, 11 or 12 or higher

**Scaling pain**: What are your worst experiences of pain? If you use 1o as the strongest exertion you have ever experienced or can think of, how strong would you say that your three worst pain experiences have been?

10   "Extremely strong—Max P" is your main point of reference. It is anchored in your previously experienced worst pain, which you just described, the "Max P".

•   Your worst pain experienced, the "Max P," may not be the highest possible level. There may be pain that is still worst. If that feeling is somewhat stronger, you will say 11 or 12. If it is much stronger, 1.5 times "Max P," you will say 15!

| | | |
|---|---|---|
| 0 | Nothing at all | "No P" |
| 0.3 | | |
| 0.5 | Extremely weak | Just noticeable |
| 1 | Very weak | |
| 1.5 | | Light |
| 2 | Weak | |
| 2.5 | | |
| 3 | Moderate | |
| 4 | | |
| 5 | Strong | Heavy |
| 6 | | |
| 7 | Very strong | |
| 8 | | |
| 9 | | |
| **10** | **Extremely strong** | **"Max P"** |
| 11 | | |
| ✦ | | |
| ● | Absolute maximum | Highest possible |

Borg CR10 scale
© Gunnar Borg, 1981, 1982, 1998

| | | |
|---|---|---|
| 0 | Nothing at all | "No P" |
| 0.3 | | |
| 0.5 | Extremely weak | Just noticeable |
| 1 | Very weak | |
| 1.5 | | Light |
| 2 | Weak | |
| 2.5 | | |
| 3 | Moderate | |
| 4 | | |
| 5 | Strong | Heavy |
| 6 | | |
| 7 | Very strong | |
| 8 | | |
| 9 | | |
| **10** | **Extremely strong** | **"Max P"** |
| 11 | | |
| ✦ | | |
| ● | Absolute maximum | Highest possible |

Borg CR10 scale
© Gunnar Borg, 1981, 1982, 1998

# Borg's CR10 Scale Instructions

**Basic instruction:** 10, "Extremely strong—Max P," is the main anchor. It is the strongest perception (P) you have ever experienced. It may be possible, however, to experience or to imagine something even stronger. Therefore, "Absolute maximum" is placed somewhat further down the scale without a fixed number and marked with a dot "•". If you perceive an intensity stronger than 10, you may use a higher number.

Start with a *verbal expression* and then choose a *number*. If your perception is "Very weak," say 1; if "Moderate," say 3; and so on. You are welcome to use half values (such as 1.5, or 3.5 or decimals, for example, 0.3, 0.8, or 2.3). It is very important that you answer what *you* perceive and not what you believe you ought to answer. Be as honest as possible and try not to overestimate or underestimate the intensities.

**Scaling perceived exertion:** We want you to rate your perceived (P) exertion, that is, how heavy and strenuous the exercise feels to you. This depends mainly on the strain and fatigue in your muscles and on your feeling of breathlessness or aches in the chest. But you must only attend to your subjective feelings and not to the physiological cues or what the actual physical load is.

| | |
|---|---|
| 1 | is "very light" like walking slowly at your own pace for several minutes. |
| 3 | is not especially hard; it feels fine, and it is no problem to continue. |
| 5 | you are tired, but you don't have any great difficulties |
| 7 | you can still go on but have to push yourself very much. You are very tired. |
| 10 | This is as hard as most people have ever experienced before in their lives. |
| • | This is "Absolute maximum," for example, 11 or 12 or higher |

**Scaling pain:** What are your worst experiences of pain? If you use 1o as the strongest exertion you have ever experienced or can think of, how strong would you say that your three worst pain experiences have been?

| | |
|---|---|
| 10 | "Extremely strong—Max P," is your main point of reference. It is anchored in your previously experienced worst pain, which you just described, the "Max P". |
| • | Your worst pain experienced, the "Max P," may not be the highest possible level. There may be pain that is still worst. If that feeling is somewhat stronger, you will say 11 or 12. If it is much stronger, 1.5 times "Max P," you will say 15! |

# Borg's CR10 Scale Instructions

**Basic instruction:** 10, "Extremely strong—Max P," is the main anchor. It is the strongest perception (P) you have ever experienced. It may be possible, however, to experience or to imagine something even stronger. Therefore, "Absolute maximum" is placed somewhat further down the scale without a fixed number and marked with a dot "•". If you perceive an intensity stronger than 10, you may use a higher number.

Start with a *verbal expression* and then choose a *number*. If your perception is "Very weak," say 1; if "Moderate," say 3; and so on. You are welcome to use half values (such as 1.5, or 3.5 or decimals, for example, 0.3, 0.8, or 2.3). It is very important that you answer what *you* perceive and not what you believe you ought to answer. Be as honest as possible and try not to overestimate or underestimate the intensities.

**Scaling perceived exertion:** We want you to rate your perceived (P) exertion, that is, how heavy and strenuous the exercise feels to you. This depends mainly on the strain and fatigue in your muscles and on your feeling of breathlessness or aches in the chest. But you must only attend to your subjective feelings and not to the physiological cues or what the actual physical load is.

| | |
|---|---|
| 1 | is "very light" like walking slowly at your own pace for several minutes. |
| 3 | is not especially hard; it feels fine, and it is no problem to continue. |
| 5 | you are tired, but you don't have any great difficulties |
| 7 | you can still go on but have to push yourself very much. You are very tired. |
| 10 | This is as hard as most people have ever experienced before in their lives. |
| • | This is "Absolute maximum," for example, 11 or 12 or higher |

**Scaling pain:** What are your worst experiences of pain? If you use 1o as the strongest exertion you have ever experienced or can think of, how strong would you say that your three worst pain experiences have been?

| | |
|---|---|
| 10 | "Extremely strong—Max P," is your main point of reference. It is anchored in your previously experienced worst pain, which you just described, the "Max P". |
| • | Your worst pain experienced, the "Max P," may not be the highest possible level. There may be pain that is still worst. If that feeling is somewhat stronger, you will say 11 or 12. If it is much stronger, 1.5 times "Max P," you will say 15! |